Everybody's Guide to
Homeopathic Medicines

Everybody's Guide to Homeopathic Medicines

Stephen Cummings, F.N.P.
Dana Ullman, M.P.H.

JEREMY P. TARCHER, INC.
Los Angeles
Disributed by Houghton Mifflin Company
Boston

Library of Congress Cataloging in Publication Data

Cummings, Stephen.
    Everybody's guide to homeopathic medicine.

    Bibliography: p. 293
    Includes index.
    1. Homeopathy—Popular works. I. Ullman, Dana.
II. Title. [DNLM: 1. Homeopathy—popular works.
WB 930 C97/e]
RX76.C94   1984   615.5'32   84-8472
ISBN 0–87477–337–7
ISBN 0–87477–324–5   (pbk.)

Jeremy P. Tarcher, Inc.
9110 Sunset Blvd.
Los Angeles, CA 90069

Text Design by Robert S. Tinnon

Manufactured in the United States of America
S   10   9   8   7   6   5   4   3   2   1

First Edition

Contents

Foreword

THE theory and practice of homeopathy is strange to those of us who are accustomed to conventional Western medicine. Dr. Samuel Hahnemann, the 19th-century founder of homeopathy, believed that remedies which, in large doses, could create a particular set of symptoms, could, in minute doses—at times so small that no molecule of the original substance remains—relieve those same symptoms.

But if homeopathy is unfamiliar, and at times seems incredible, it is not uncongenial. We look hopefully for medicines that offer answers to the chronic conditions afflicting so many of us and eluding the curative reach of conventional medicine. We want drugs that have fewer debilitating side effects. And we sense the rightness of a healing system which conceives of all symptoms as parts of a larger whole, which appears to stimulate the body's natural healing force, rather than attack its enemies. Homeopathy seems to work with us, not on us.

Everybody's Guide to Homeopathic Medicines is an enormously useful introduction to the theory and practice of homeopathy. It briefly traces the homeopathic movement from its heyday in mid-nineteenth-century America (when one in five American physicians in urban areas were homeopaths), through its eclipse by the American Medical Association, to its remarkable renaissance in the 1970s and 80s. It provides an introduction to the theory of homeopathic prescribing and casetaking. It offers a useful distillation of the extensive and usually overwhelming *materia medica* (the catalog of homeopathic medicines and their specific characteristics), a glossary of unfamiliar terms, and a list of references.

The heart of the book is, however, a series of chapters on common ailments and their homeopathic treatments. This is appropriate; homeopathy has always been a practical and a participatory discipline. These chapters, with their descriptions of symptoms and their matching remedies, permit any careful reader to select the appropriate remedy—for fever, colds, skin problems, aches and pains, and other minor but distressing ailments. They invite us to participate in the evolution of the discipline, to see for ourselves if homeopathy works.

In presenting the material, the authors are careful to delineate the arena in which lay or self prescription is to be used. Each chapter makes clear those situations which are "Beyond Home Care" and which require consultation with a health care professional. This is a valuable service—at once responsible and adventurous. Responsible because it admonishes practitioners to appreciate the range of illness with which they can safely deal, and adventurous because it helps reconcile homeopathic and conventional health care practice.

I believe the renaissance of homeopathy will continue. I know that many of those whom I and my homeopathic colleagues have treated have become enthusiastic advocates and students of homeopathy. At the same time, interest among young physicians and medical students is increasing. Cummings's and Ullman's book will provide an entry point for those who would like to experience the challenge of homeopathic casetaking and treatment. It will whet the appetite of those who may eventually make the theoretical formulations and undertake the research which will help us to come to terms with this little-understood but fascinating approach to health care.

James S. Gordon, M.D.
Georgetown University School of Medicine

Acknowledgments

We would like to acknowledge the following people who reviewed all or part of this book: Maesimund Panos, M.D., Edward C. Whitmont, M.D., Randy Neustaedter, Jeff Gould, M.D., Louis Klein, Jacquelyn Wilson, M.D., Bob Stewart, Margaret Macasland, Fred Cagle, and Della Desrosiers. Janice Gallagher, our editor, did a phenomenal job bringing order to our initially massive manuscript and deserves special credit for making this book usable and understandable.

Heartfelt thanks also to our many friends and colleagues who helped us in one way or another: Jayme Canton, Liz Gregory, Greg Manteuffel, M.D., Ina Gordon, Diana Jackson, Nancy Herrick, David Anderson, M.D., Peggy Chipkin, Christine Ciavarella, Jack Guralnik, M.D., Ray Rosenthal, M.D., Kathleen Haley, Corey Weinstein, M.D., Carole, Lisa, and Jason Morison, Marshall Cummings, Robert Bruce Moody, Sally and Sarah Aldinger, Alan Solares, Selden Cummings, Celia Cummings, Richard Grossinger, David Hoskinson, Marc Lappe, Harris Coulter, Burt Linnetz, Don Gerrard, Chris Mole, Jocelyn Stoller, Arnold Whitridge and Dannon Lahey.

Dana Ullman: It is wonderful to have a father who is loving and supportive. It is a special privilege that he, as a physician and pediatrician, was also able to review our manuscript to assure that the book provided the most up-to-date medical information. My mother's continual love and support has also been inspiring to me in my work and in helping me be the person that I am.

Why and How
to Use This Book

H OMEOPATHY is a 200-year-old medical system you can use at home to help treat family members with a wide spectrum of acute health problems. It offers a way to gently stimulate our inner healing resources through recognizing and reinforcing the adaptive reactions of our natural defense processes. By choosing the correct, individually suited homeopathic medicine from the plant, mineral, animal, or chemical kingdom, you can successfully stimulate the body's own defenses. Following our instructions, you can complement your family's efforts toward good health with these safe, natural medicines that provide an effective, inexpensive alternative to conventional medicine.

The best reason to use homeopathic medicines in self-care is that they work. When the medicines are prescribed correctly, they act rapidly, deeply, and curatively, stimulating the body's defenses, rather than simply suppressing symptoms.

Homeopathic medicines are exceptional, as they can so greatly enhance deep healing without the harmful side effects so commonly caused by conventional medicines. What's more, the homeopathic medicines cost much less than conventional drugs. As violinist Yehudi Menuhin, president of the Hahnemann Society in the United Kingdom—one of the largest homeopathic organizations in the U.K.—once said, "Homeopathy is one of the rare medical approaches which carries no penalties—only benefits."

Homeopathy works effectively in treating people with a wide variety of acute and chronic problems, including infectious disease, allergies, gynecological conditions, digestive problems, skin diseases, and even psychological and genetic disorders. The scope of effective homeopathic treatment is broad, but this book will not teach you to treat *all* health problems that you or your family can experience. The proper role of homeopathic medicine at home is in the treatment of people with mild-to-moderate acute conditions. Acute conditions are self-limiting accidents or illnesses that are short in duration, have a generally predictable course, and resolve without significant aftereffects. Using homeopathic treatment at home, you can speed the healing of a wide variety of conditions. Of course, some acute conditions require medical supervision, and we alert you to potentially serious symptoms in the "Beyond Home Care" section of each chapter in part 2 of this book. Homeopathy may nevertheless help minimize the severity of the problem and speed healing in even these cases.

Chronic diseases, in contrast to acute ones, are long in duration, degenerative in nature, and do not tend to resolve spontaneously. Such illnesses are complex, and their care requires a great deal of knowledge of the medical sciences and of homeopathy. People with chronic disease need the care of an experienced homeopath, who can often help them feel stronger, experience less pain, and slow down the degenerative process.

Our book is divided into three main sections. Part 1 covers homeopathic history, principles, and practical methodology. We urge you to read this introductory material carefully before you undertake home treatment. To be consistently successful, you must understand the philosophies and principles that are the foundation of the homeopathic method.

In part 2 we individually cover a wide variety of acute conditions for which home care with homeopathic medicines is often appropriate. Our discussion of each condition in these "clinical" chapters is organized into several sections: a general description of the condition, advice on simple home care measures, a list of possible homeopathic medicines and the symptoms each covers that are relevant to the condition, and "Beyond Home Care," a summary of warning signs that require professional care.

Part 3 consists of the *materia medica,* in which most of the medicines included in the clinical chapters are listed and their general characteristics described. Each medicine has a set of symptoms common to all conditions for which it may be properly used. The information in part 3 is complementary to the descriptions of the specific symptoms in part 2; part 3 gives you more information about the medicines you are considering and helps you choose among them.

It is our greatest hope that this book serve as the beginning of your involvement in homeopathy. Therefore, in part 4 we provide you with listings of homeopathic books, organizations, and pharmacies to help you obtain more information about homeopathic medicine.

The Chinese believe that the best doctors use no medicines and, instead, heal by giving guidance on how to live properly. Strictly speaking, homeopathy is a system of giving medicines, and even natural medicines can only temporarily improve symptoms caused by continued exposure to personal or societal health stress (influences homeopaths call "obstacles to cure"). That said, if you are willing to put your powers of observation and judgment to use—and if you're treating others, your communications skills as well—you'll receive the most satisfying rewards by using homeopathic medicines at home: a greater understanding of you and your family's health and the knowledge that you're not only feeling better but becoming truly healthier as well.

PART
1

Understanding
Homeopathic
Medicine

CHAPTER 1

The Science of Homeopathy

In the late 1700s, homeopathy emerged as a highly systematic medical science through the efforts of German physician Samuel Hahnemann. Prior to developing homeopathic science, Hahnemann had been an esteemed physician and chemist. He was the personal physician to members of the German royalty and the author of one of the most respected texts on chemistry in his day. Despite his successes, he left his own orthodox medical practice; he felt he was doing more harm than good with the routine use of bloodletting, poisonous doses of mercury and arsenic, and the other often harmful medical practices that were in vogue.

Hahnemann was a scholar of numerous languages, and because he had a family to support, he resorted to translating various medical and literary texts. While translating a work by William Cullen, a leading physiologist of the time, Hahnemann was startled by the author's claim that the bitter and astringent properties of Peruvian bark, which contains quinine, accounted for its effectiveness in treating malaria. Hahnemann proved Cullen wrong by preparing an even more bitter and astringent mixture that was useless against malaria.

Hahnemann decided to test the physiological effects of Peruvian bark by taking small doses himself. His body eventually reacted to the drug. To his surprise, he developed symptoms very similar to those of malaria. Hahnemann wondered whether the curative power of Peruvian bark resulted from its capacity to create symptoms similar to those of the disease.

By studying the records of accidental poisonings from other commonly used medicines of his time, such as mercury, arsenic, belladonna, and silver nitrate, and by testing these poisons on himself and others, he found that in overdose the "medicines" caused symptoms similar to those of the illnesses for which they were used. Mercury, used to treat syphilis, could cause syphilislike ulcers. Arsenic and belladonna were known to create certain types of fever and were given as medicines for fevers. Silver nitrate, applied for eye inflammation, caused severe irritation and discharge from the eyes.

The Law of Similars: The Basic Principle of Homeopathy

To like things like, whatever one may ail; there is certain help.

—Johann Wolfgang Goethe, *Faust*

Hahnemann coined the Latin phrase *similia similibus curentur* ("let likes be cured with likes") to describe his discovery that substances in small dose stimulate the organism to heal that which they cause in overdose. He termed the medical system based on this principle "homeopathy" from the Greek words *homoios* for "similar" and *pathos* for "suffering" or "disease." This principle, most commonly known as the "law of similars," states that any substance which can cause symptoms when given to healthy people can help to heal those who are experiencing similar symptoms.

The law of similars has been used throughout history and throughout the world, both in and out of health care (Boyd 1936; Coulter 1975, 1977, 1982; Grossinger, 1982). In the fourth century B.C. Hippocrates wrote, "Through the like, disease is produced, and through the application of the like it is cured." Paracelsus, a well-known, fifteenth-century physician and alchemist, used the law of similars extensively in his practice and his writings. He affirmed, "You there bring together the same anatomy of the herbs and the same anatomy of the illness into one order. This simile gives you an understanding of the way in which you shall heal" (Coulter 1975: 432).

Some of the *similia* concept has a place in conventional medicine as well. Since the time of Edward Jenner, small doses of agents that cause illness been given to immunize patients against diseases. Radiation is a cancer treatment, though it can cause cancer. Ritalin, an amphetamine-like drug, is given to hyperactive children. Gold is used to treat some types of arthritis despite the fact that it can cause joint pain. Although these and numerous other medical treatments are reminiscent of the fundamental principle of homeopathy, none of them obey the other essential tenets of homeopathic practice: individualization of the drug to the person's total physical and psychological characteristics, the use of the single medicine at the minimum dose, and the unique homeopathic pharmaceutical process.

There has been some technical research in physics, biology, biochemistry, and other natural sciences to determine how the law of similars works (Barnard and Stephenson 1967, 1969; Stephenson 1955, 1961, 1967; Tiller 1979). Though important, a theoretical or technical explanation of this phenomenon is secondary to the success homeopathic medicines have brought to millions of homeopathic patients and practitioners.

Symptoms As Defenses: Appreciating the Body's Healing Process

Hahnemann's observation that a substance that can mimic symptoms helps cure a person revealed a revolutionary understanding of symptoms. Instead of assuming that symptoms represent illogical, improper, or unhealthy responses of the body and that they should be treated, controlled, and suppressed, Hahnemann learned that symptoms are positive, adaptive responses to the variety of stresses the body experiences. Symptoms represent the body's best effort to heal itself. Hence, instead of suppressing symptoms, therapies should stimulate the body's defenses to complete the curative process.

This understanding of illness was not without precedent in Western medical history. A long tradition in Western culture, dating from Hippocrates in 400 B.C., has been that symptoms benefit the organism by dealing with the stresses impinging on it (Coulter 1975, 1977, 1982). The ancient phrase *vis medicatrix naturae*, meaning "the healing power of nature," refers directly to the human organism's dynamic and powerful capacity to protect and heal itself.

Present-day physicians and scientists commonly acknowledge this "wisdom of the body." Hans Selye, internationally respected physician and scientist, noted, "Disease is not mere surrender to attack but also fight for health; unless there is a fight, there is no disease. . . . Disease is not just suffering, but a fight to maintain the homeostatic balance of our tissues, despite damage" (1978: 12–13).

In this context, symptoms are not the disease. Symptoms *accompany* disease. Symptoms are evidence of disease. But treating symptoms is like killing the messenger for bringing bad news. In fact, by treating symptoms, you are suppressing the body's natural responses and inhibiting the healing process.

As a systematic observer of nature and healing, Hahnemann was savvy enough to recognize that the body makes amazing and impressive efforts to heal itself, but that it is not always strong enough to complete the healing process. It often needs a catalyst to stimulate its defenses, particularly when battling serious acute infectious disease, chronic illness, or genetic disorders. With the law of similars, Hahnemann developed a highly systematic method to individualize the choice of the right catalyst by prescribing a substance that imitates the body's defenses.

Hahnemann strongly criticized conventional medical therapies of his day that simply suppressed symptoms. He frequently noted that the many "successes" of conventional medical treatments were only temporary and often harmful, since the symptoms often returned or more threatening symptoms manifested as the body sought to reestablish its internal harmony.

As Nobel Prize–winning scientist René Dubos said, "Western medicine will become scientific only when physicians and their patients have learned to manage the forces of the body and the mind that operate in *vis medicatrix naturae*." Homeopathic medicine *is* this scientific method.

The Homeopathic Provings:
Assessing Toxic and Therapeutic
Properties of Medicines

Most drug experimentation conducted by orthodox medical researchers has been performed on sick people, on animals, or in laboratories. As an ever-innovative contributor to medical science, Hahnemann was the first to recommend giving medicinal drugs to healthy people to assess their physiological properties. These experiments, called "provings," involve giving the person small doses of the single substance on a daily basis until symptoms are elicited. The dose used is extremely small and is selected according to previous knowledge of the toxic properties of the potential medicine. Careful observations and records are made of the symptoms that occur. Each substance creates a variety of physical, emotional, and mental symptoms, unique to that substance.

Initially, Hahnemann used mostly herbs and heavy metals like mercury and arsenic for his provings, the drugs employed by orthodox practitioners of his day. Later he tested various herbs used in European folk medicine, and other homeopaths have since "proven" herbal medicines of many regions, and many other mineral- and animal-derived substances.

The homeopathic provings provide the experimental basis for learning what symptoms a substance causes and thus, according to the law of similars, what it cures. The provings allow the practitioner to individualize the choice of a medicine according to the totality of the patient's symptoms.

The detailed records of the symptoms produced during the provings are compiled in reference books known as *materia medica.* The *materia medica* (Latin for "materials of medicine") list the medicines used in homeopathy and describe in detail the specific psychological and physical symptoms of each medicine. *Repertories* are indices to the information found in the *materia medica* and catalog thousands of symptoms. Under each symptom listed are all relevant homeopathic medicines, those medicines known to cause the symptom, and thus those that may be indicated in treating a person with that symptom.

Although most of the provings were done in the 1800s and early 1900s, the American Institute of Homeopathy started a program of reproving the medicines in the 1940s. This effort ended when the institute discovered that the medicines caused the same symptoms previously listed. The homeopathic reference books are as valuable today as when they were first published.

The Totality of Symptoms

As far back as 180 years ago, long before the term "holistic health" was coined, homeopaths recognized the inseparability of body and mind. Homeopaths have always stressed the importance of assessing the totality of the person.

Hahnemann found that many of the substances he tested in provings provoked common symptoms such as fever, diarrhea, cough, restlessness, irritability, and so on. Still, each created a unique overall pattern of physiological and psychological change. Hahnemann determined he needed to match the total pattern of a substance's toxic symptoms with all the sick person's own symptoms to effect a cure. These matchings had to be precise and individualized. Matching only a few common symptoms or prescribing medicines routinely—giving Peruvian bark to everyone with malaria, for instance—was not effective.

The homeopathic definition of the term "symptom" encompasses the physical and psychological, the obvious and subtle, the common and the unusual. Even if the person has a main symptom that is causing much discomfort, the homeopath must also assess all other physical and psychological symptoms. Characteristic emotional states, changes in the person's energy level, sensitivity to heat or cold, and numerous other factors must all be considered.

The assumption is that no matter what combination of conditions, complaints, and sufferings the patient experiences at any one time, all are the manifestation of a single "disease," an internal physiological disorder that is unique to the individual. The homeopath believes that no one organ of the body can be sick without affecting the person as a whole. Therefore, all symptoms must be taken into account; all are part of the body's effort to heal. It is crucial to understand that, in spite of the homeopath's desire to know all the minute details of the patient's symptoms, he or she does not *treat* symptoms. Instead the symptoms guide the homeopath to the medicine that can best stimulate the person's defenses.

Just as no isolated part of the body can be sick alone, the various recurrent symptoms people experience throughout their lives evolve from one enduring "constitutional" weakness. Such an underlying constitutional weakness or susceptibility is best treated by an experienced homeopath, whether the prominent symptoms in evidence are chronic or acute flare-ups of a recurrent problem. This approach is called *constitutional homeopathy*. Often, however, the most pronounced symptoms of an acute illness are the body's response to a specific set of acute stresses—infection, psychological stress, exposure to extremes of weather or to toxic substances, lack of sleep, and such. During true acute illnesses, the body mounts a strong healing defense against these particular acute stresses and devotes most of its healing resources to the effort. These are the illnesses that can be treated at home by the lay homeopath, who can choose the medicines on the basis of the prominent acute symptoms alone.

The Single Medicine

A homeopath does not prescribe one medicine for a person's headache, another for her stomachache, and another for her depression. The use of a single medicine at a time is a basic principle of classical homeopathy. As we've said, the homeopath assumes that, although a person may have numerous physical and psychological symptoms, he or she has only one disease, an underlying susceptibility. Using the one medicine right for that time in the person's life, whether the condition is acute or chronic, effectively stimulates the person's natural defense system, helps heal the current illness, and raises the general level of health.

Although sometimes effective, *mixtures* of medicines cannot be used according to the law of similars on the basis of provings of the individual substances they contain. The new mixture may have some characteristics of each component substance but also some unique to the mixture. Its indications are unknown until a separate homeopathic proving is performed. More details about the use of combination medicines are provided in the section "Variations of Homeopathic Practice" later in this chapter.

One value of the single medicine in healing is that its use helps the practitioner and patient know the effect of treatment. Research has shown that during a stay in a hospital patients receive an average of nine different medicines. The side effects of individual drugs are often startling enough, but the unknown, synergistic effects of numerous medicines given together to an already disordered physiology may be frightening.

The Minimum Number of Doses

An essential precept in homeopathy is the principle of the minimum number of doses. Hahnemann strongly believed in the importance of this principle and felt that a person's inherent healing powers were so strong that only a small stimulus was needed to begin the healing process. In fact, Hahnemann and numerous other homeopaths have asserted that once the healing process begins it is best to do nothing more but let the process continue in its own way. Another dose of medicine may be required at some future time, but classical homeopaths are adamant about prescribing no other medicine or dose until the first has completed its action. Since the medicines act as a catalyst to the body's own defenses, continual repetition is not needed. In the treatment of chronic illnesses, months or sometimes years may pass before reintroducing a medicine. A special benefit of the minimum-dose principle is its discouraging the obsession with treatment in the process of finding the best, most efficient, and deepest-acting medicine.

The Potentized Dose: Homeopathy's Pharmaceutical Process

When Samuel Hahnemann first began applying the law of similars in his medical practice, he obtained impressive results. However, he noted that patients sometimes developed toxic symptoms as a result of an overdose of the medicine. Hahnemann began to experiment with the size of the dose to see how little medicine he could give to still cause a sustained healing response. After years of rigorous study he found a method of diluting substances that kept the toxic properties at a minimum while the potential to cure was magnified. He called this pharmaceutical process "potentization."

Potentization consists of a process of successive dilution. If the medicine is soluble, 1 part is diluted in 99 parts of water or alcohol, and the mixture is mixed vigorously by striking the bottle against a firm surface. If the medicine is insoluble it is finely ground, or *triturated*, in the same proportions with powdered lactose (milk sugar). One part of the diluted medicine is then diluted again in the same manner, and the process is repeated as many times as necessary to achieve the desired final dilution strength. The most common strengths have been diluted as often as 3, 6, 30, 200, 1000, 10,000, 50,000, or 100,000 times. The medicines that are diluted 1 part to 99 parts are called *centesimal* potencies and may be labeled 6c, 30c, and so on, though often the *c* is omitted. Sometimes the dilution factor is 1 part medicine to 9 parts dilutant, and these *decimal* potencies are always labeled 6x, 30x, and so on.

By convention, a medicine that has been diluted fewer times than another is considered a lower potency. This is a relative distinction, but usually medicines diluted fifteen times or less (15c, 15x, or lower) are referred to as low potencies, while those diluted more than this are considered high potencies (30c and higher).

Potentization is different from simple dilution. Homeopaths have found that the medicines do not work if they are simply diluted repeatedly without vigorous shaking or if they are just diluted in vast amounts of liquid. Nor do the medicines work if they are only vigorously shaken. It is the combined process of dilution and vigorous shaking that makes the medicine effective, when the symptoms of the medicine are similar to those of the ill person.

That tiny amounts of various substances can cause significant physiological changes is not new to medical science. A milligram of acetylcholine dissolved in 500,000 gallons of blood has long been known to lower the blood pressure of a cat, and even smaller amounts affect the beat of a frog's heart (Cottell, 1930: 256). Florey, the co-discoverer of penicillin, reported in 1943 that pure penicillin can inhibit the development of sensitive microorganisms in the laboratory at dilutions of 1:50,000,000 to 1:100,000,000. The human body manufactures only 50 to 100 millionths of a gram of thyroid hormone per day, and the concentration of free thyroid hormone in normal blood is just 1 part per 10,000 million parts of blood plasma (Evans 1968: 1493–1494). Yet this hormone is a powerful regulator of metabolic rate.

There have been numerous other experiments in the fields of botany, zoology, bacteriology, and physics (Stephenson 1955; Coulter 1981) that attest to the power of microdoses, including homeopathic potencies more dilute than 12c. Double-blind clinical and laboratory studies have also provided evidence that the medicines act even though the dose is infinitesimal. One study in the *British Journal of Clinical Pharmacology* showed the effectiveness of homeopathic medicines in treating people with rheumatoid arthritis. Over 80% of the patients who received a homeopathic medicine experienced improvement in their arthritic symptoms, while only about 20% of the patients who received a placebo had similar improvement. It is interesting to note that both physicians involved in the experiment obtained a similar rate of improvement, indicating that the medicine rather than the practitioner played the primary role in the therapeutic success.

Other well-controlled double-blind studies have shown the effectiveness of the homeopathic medicines in treating people exposed to mustard gas (Paterson 1941) and rats exposed to lead (Fisher 1983). Dr. Harris L. Coulter's *Homoeopathic Science and Modern Medicine* (1981), Dana Ullman's *Monograph on Homeopathic Research,* (1980), and Boiron Laboratories' *Aspects of Research in Homeopathy* (1983) have provided further evidence of the efficacy of the microdose.

Homeopaths have found, in fact, that generally the more a substance is potentized, the deeper it acts, the longer it acts, and the fewer number of doses are required in treatment. Although the higher potencies—those that have been diluted and shaken more— are generally more powerful than the lower potencies, all have a place in clinical practice. Since the higher potencies are particularly powerful, they must be used very judiciously. Homeopaths recommend that laypeople and beginning students of homeopathy not prescribe potencies higher than 30c.

Potentization is probably the most controversial part of the homeopathic method. Most scientists believe that no medicine diluted more than the 12c potency could have any biochemical effect, since it is improbable that any molecules of the original substance remain.

Many observers suggest that, in fact, the benefits of homeopathic treatment are due to the placebo effect. Evidence to the contrary is the impressive clinical successes homeopaths have had treating serious infectious illnesses such as cholera, yellow fever, and whooping cough. Homeopathic literature also records many successes in the treatment of seriously ill infants and all kinds of animals, presumably not responsive to the placebo effect. In addition, carefully conducted provings using the high potencies have produced patterns of symptoms similar to provings done with the low potencies.

Homeopathic medicines thus have physiological activity, though we still do not understand how or why they act. Practicing homeopaths use the medicines because they work and await further research for the explanation.

Hering's Laws of Cure

Homeopaths define health as a state of freedom existing on three interrelated levels: the physical, the emotional, and the mental. A healthy person experiences physical vitality and freedom from physiological malfunction, emotional peace and freedom of expression, and mental clarity with creativity. The most serious symptoms affect the deeper, more vital parts of the person. Evaluation of our overall state of health, according to the homeopath, depends most on our mental state, next on our emotional state, and third on our physical state.

A homeopath is not content to hear that the symptom for which the patient originally came to be treated has improved. The practitioner needs to know what else has changed, for better or worse, and whether the person's overall vitality has increased or decreased. If, for instance, a skin problem has improved but a chest infection has developed, the homeopath may conclude that the therapy has actually made the person worse.

Experience with homeopathic treatment has shown that, following the administration of the correct medicine, symptoms on the deeper levels improve while those on more external levels often temporarily worsen. It has come to be expected that the cure will progress from inside out, and this progress can be used to validate the success of treatment. Details of the important changes in posttreatment symptoms were codified by Constantine Hering, a German homeopath who emigrated to the United States in the 1830s and who is considered the father of American homeopathy. The three general principles of the homeopathic healing process are known as Hering's laws of cure.

According to the first of Hering's laws, healing progresses from the deepest part of the organism—the mental and emotional levels and the vital organs—to the external parts, such as the skin and extremities. A cure is in progress when a person's psychological symptoms lessen and the physical symptoms increase (so long as the physical symptoms are not severely pathological). Eventually, as this healing moves outward, even the superficial symptoms are alleviated. On the other hand, if physical symptoms improve but the psychological state worsens, the person's state of health is thought to be deteriorating.

Within each of the three broad levels of the defense system, symptoms that affect more vital functions are the deepest and most threatening to health. George Vithoulkas, a respected contemporary homeopath, has outlined the varying depths of symptoms from each level (1980; 24), in descending order of depth, symptoms and their impact on one's state of health.

Physical	Emotional	Mental
Brain ailments	Suicidal depression	Complete confusion
Heart ailments	Apathy	Destructive delirium
Endocrine ailments	Sadness	Paranoid ideas
Liver ailments	Anguish	Delusions
Lung ailments	Phobias	Lethargy
Kidney ailments	Anxiety	Dullness
Bone ailments	Irritability	Lack of
Muscle ailments	Dissatisfaction	concentration
Skin ailments		Forgetfulness
		Absentmindedness

The exact location of these symptoms in the table is not as important as the outline's use as a guide for evaluating the patient's progress according to Hering's first law.

Hering's second law states that, as healing progresses, symptoms appear and disappear in the reverse of their original chronological order of appearance. Homeopaths have observed that consistently their patients reexperience symptoms from past conditions. The time during which the patient suffered from these conditions may range from six months to ten or twenty years before the present treatment. These observations, of course, pertain more to patients being treated for chronic conditions, but even during an acute illness a retracing of the development of the symptoms may be noticeable after the medicine is given.

According to Hering's third law, healing progresses from the upper to the lower parts of the body. For instance, a person is considered to be on the mend if the arthritic pain in his neck has decreased although he now has pain in the finger joints.

As the symptoms change in accordance with a Hering law, it is common for individual symptoms to become worse than they had been before treatment. These aggravations are welcomed by the knowledgeable homeopath, provided there is corresponding improvement in the symptoms on deeper levels, of more recent onset, and higher on the body. If healing is truly in progress, the patient feels stronger and generally better in spite of the aggravation. Before long, the symptoms of the aggravation pass and leave the person healthier on all levels.

Hering's laws are extremely valuable tools in the holistic assessment of health, for they provide a way to evaluate the person's total state of health, not only the person's main complaint. Sometimes, however, the three guidelines of Hering's laws as observed in a patient may not conform to the classic pattern. For instance, the symptoms may move from within outward, in accordance with the first law, but also travel upward, violating the third law. Whenever the progress of healing is difficult to interpret, the final judgement depends on whether the person experiences an overall increase in freedom. An apparent violation of one law may be insignificant if the symptoms that arise are minor. It is most important that the other laws are observed and the person's general state improves.

Homeopaths are not the only practitioners who have observed

the existence of Hering's laws. Acupuncturists have witnessed aspects of these laws for thousands of years. Psychotherapists and healers utilizing various natural therapies have also noticed this phenomenon.

The main use of Hering's laws for you will be in home treatment situations. You'll want to know whether the medicine you have given is helping. That the medicine is working is usually obvious. In acute situations the homeopathic healing response is usually rapid and complete, and the progress of symptoms as it follows the laws often will be too rapid to notice. Whenever you are in doubt about a person's response, however, consider the changes in symptoms in light of Hering's laws.

The Homeopathic View of Infectious Disease

Most commonly, the illnesses you will treat at home with homeopathy are the acute infectious diseases. An infectious disease is the disruption of normal body function that occurs when a microorganism enters the body, multiplies, and thrives where it is not normally present.* The signs and symptoms of the illness result from the interaction between the the germ, which injures or poisons the tissue, and the person's inherent physiological defenses, which respond to the infection.

Although many today think of homeopathy as useful mostly for psychosomatic conditions or other chronic problems, the rapid spread of the treatment in the early 1800s resulted from its superior record in fighting deadly epidemics of cholera, typhoid, scarlet fever, yellow fever, and other infectious diseases. You won't be treating such serious illnesses at home, but homeopathy remains an effective therapy for people with all types of infections.

---

*Further evidence that Hahnemann was ahead of his time is the fact that in 1832, at least thirty years before scientists recognized the existence of germs, he noted that the cholera epidemic was due to a "brood of . . . excessively minute, invisible, living creatures" (1852).

Homeopaths do not assume that germs are the primary cause of infections. In order to determine the "cause" of an infectious disease, it is necessary to take into account both the virulence of the infecting agent *and* the resistance of the person's defense system. This broader view of infectious disease explains how, in the same environment and exposed to the same germs, some people get sick and others do not. Biologists and homeopaths refer to these phenomena as "states of susceptibility" and "host resistance."

Indeed, homeopaths see the presence of microbes as the *result* of disease, and they understand the "disease" to be the preexisting susceptibility of the person to infection—the constitutional weakness previously discussed. For instance, that a throat culture shows *Streptococcus* bacteria are growing in a child's throat does not necessarily mean the germ *caused* the illness. The problem is that the child's defense system is not as strong as it could be, and this weakness created an environment conducive to the growth of bacteria.

In fact, strep bacteria often live harmlessly in the throats of people who have no symptoms and who are resistant to the infection. Medical tests frequently show that individuals have various bacteria, viruses, and other pathological agents in their bodies yet are not ill. It is usually only when the person's defenses are significantly weakened by some type of stress, whether it be malnutrition, lack of exercise, mental or emotional stress, or exposure to chemical or environmental dangers, that the pathological agents are able to multiply easily enough to make the body vulnerable to disease.

Certainly some microbes are so virulent that few individuals can build resistance to them. Widespread epidemics have often been related to social upheavals, malnutrition, poor hygiene, and the like, but in some cases they have decimated apparently healthy populations. Epidemics and virulent infections aside, the overall resistance of the person and his or her exposure to stress are of primary importance in dealing with ordinary illnesses.

The homeopathic approach to infectious disease assumes that most people have sufficiently strong physiological resources to overcome infecting organisms and restore good health. Homeopathic medicines strengthen and rally these inherent resources, and those treated homeopathically not only recover faster but become more resistant to other infections as well.

Since homeopathic medicines do not kill germs directly, the agent associated with the illness, be it bacteria, virus, fungi, or other microbe, makes little difference. The sometimes difficult process of diagnosis and the inability of conventional therapies to treat viral conditions are not impediments to homeopathic treatment. No germ will remain a major problem for the person whose defenses are sufficiently strong.

Most medical research concerning infectious disease has focused on how to kill germs or inhibit their growth rather than how to stimulate the body's own defenses. Antibiotics, the main group of drugs used to combat bacterial infection, may help rid the body of certain bacteria, but they don't change the various factors that led to the infection. As Dr. Marc Lappe, pathologist and associate professor at University of California at Berkeley, writes in his powerful book *Germs That Won't Die* (1982: 173), "A basic truism of antibiotic treatment is that it will not work under most circumstances unless the body can mount its own attack against invading bacteria." In fact, the person for whom antibiotics are prescribed may become more susceptible to further infections if the antibiotic inhibits the growth of beneficial bacteria, those that aid digestion and protect the skin and mucous membranes. Resistance to infection may even be lowered when certain patients experience side effects caused by antibiotics. Dr. Lappe cites a recent study that showed certain antibiotics actually depress the body's immune responses (1982: 178).

The emergence of microorganisms resistant to antibiotics poses another problem with using these drugs. Harvard University professor Walter Gilbert has stated, "There may be a time down the road when 80% to 90% of infections will be resistant to all known antibiotics" (Cave, *Time*, August 17, 1981).

Despite such drawbacks, antibiotics can literally be lifesaving when serious infections of vital organs occur. Most infections, however, are not life-or-death situations, so when you or your child has an illness that might respond to antibiotic treatment, deciding whether or not to use antibiotics may be difficult. You should consult your health practitioner to discuss such factors as the severity of the illness, the person's vitality, and the possible alternatives, including homeopathy.

If you or your child receives antibiotic treatment for an infectious illness, we strongly recommend you follow the prescription's instructions carefully. Take the drug for the entire time prescribed, even if symptoms diminish rapidly. Even if you are receiving antibiotic treatment, we recommend you take an appropriate homeopathic medicine concurrently. While antibiotics may interfere with the action of the homeopathic medicine to some degree, we have often observed that people being treated with antibiotics tend to improve more rapidly after administration of the homeopathic remedy. People often continue to have symptoms of their illness even after the antibiotic treatment is complete, and when this occurs homeopathic treatment is again appropriate.

Variations of Homeopathic Practice

Many practitioners use nonclassical variations of homeopathy, and some of these approaches have become especially popular: combination or polypharmacy homeopathy refers to the use of more than one medicine at a time. This type of homeopathy is commonly practiced in Europe, and combinations of homeopathic medicines meant for home use are appearing with increasing frequency in health food stores and even retail pharmacies and supermarkets in America. The combination medicines include mixtures of low potency dose of the most often-used medicines for specific conditions. Classical homeopaths assert that combination medicines should have experimental provings done to determine their specific usage, since substances once mixed together acquire different properties from the individual components'. They claim that the indiscriminate use of many medicines can disorder a person's case and make it more difficult to find the correct medicine. As with those who use low potency medicines, those who use combination medicines usually do not pay much attention to the person's psychological characteristics. Also, the low-potency combination medicine generally requires frequent repetition, and its curative powers are generally less complete than those of the single, correct medicine.

Despite these criticisms, many European physicians and American consumers hail the effectiveness of the combination medicines. We look forward to systematic studies that clarify their value.

"Cell salts," also called the "twelve tissue salts," are commonly used medicines often thought of as being similar to homeopathy. They were developed by a German physician, Dr. W. H. Schussler, in the 1870s, who found these simple mineral substances to be the most abundant constituents of cremated human remains. Schussler's theory was that these simple minerals are largely responsible for harmonious function of physiological processes and that disease results when the body is deficient in these minerals or when their metabolism is disordered. He thought that such problems could be corrected by supplying the appropriate mineral, homeopathically prepared.

These theories of disease appear antiquated and simplistic in the light of modern understanding of physiology. While minerals and their proper balance are vitally important to homeostatic processes, there are many complex physiologic systems that depend as well on thousands of biochemicals, not simply twelve inorganic minerals.

Although the cell salt theory may not be accurate, the potentized cell salts certainly have effects on organisms. All cell salts are used by classical homeopaths for the specific physical and psychological symptoms that they create in provings. Most users of cell salts, however, prescribe them on very limited physical symptoms. Also, since many cell salt users take more than one medicine at a time, the criticisms previously stated of such practice are applicable here too.

The Bach Flower remedies were developed by a British bacteriologist and homeopath named Edward Bach. By observing ailing animals' licking the dew from flowers, Bach intuited how each flower influences different emotional states and developed his system of thirty-eight flower remedies for thirty-eight different emotional states. These remedies are based only on a person's psychological symptoms. The person's physical symptoms do not play any role in determining the remedy. Also, distinct from homeopathy, the Bach remedies are not prescribed according to information obtained in provings. Usually more than one remedy is prescribed at a time, and frequent repetition of the medicine is recommended. Some people who use the Bach remedies claim subtle or more obvious improvements in their psychological state. Only in rare situations do people note improvement of physical symptoms.

Historical Notes and the Status of Homeopathy Today

Although rejected by the medical establishment of the nineteenth century, homeopathy spread rapidly throughout Europe and then to the United States in the years following Hahnemann's announcement of his discoveries, largely because of its medical successes with the dread epidemic illnesses. In 1900 a comparison of mortality rates among homeopathic and conventional medical patients throughout the United States and Europe showed that between two to eight times as many homeopathic patients with life-threatening infectious diseases survived as compared with those receiving conventional medical care of the day (Bradford 1900).

The history of homeopathic medicine in America is fascinating. Few people, including doctors, are aware that the first national medical association in the United States was the American Institute of Homeopathy, founded in 1844. By the turn of the century fully 20%–25% of all physicians in urban areas identified themselves as homeopaths. There were 22 homeopathic medical schools, and over 100 homeopathic hospitals. Many well-known people were patrons of homeopathy, including William James, Harriet Beecher Stowe, Henry Wadsworth Longfellow, John D. Rockefeller, Louisa May Alcott, and Daniel Webster. William Cullen Bryant, noted journalist and poet, was the president of the Homeopathic Medical Society of New York City and County.

Since the turn of the century, however, homeopathy declined to the point that few people outside the health professions had even heard the word. Some of the reasons for this decline included: (1) Strong opposition from the AMA. The AMA Code of Ethics prohibited members from consulting with homeopathic physicians, even if conventional medical treatments were failing. Orthodox physicians influenced legislation that limited homeopathic training and practice. (2) Recent advances in modern medicine. Though the orthodox treatments of Hahnemann's day were largely ineffective and often caused immediate suffering or even death, the twentieth century saw a rapid growth in treatments that were at least superficially successful. Powerful pain-killing drugs and other suppressive medicines seemed to work magically, though they merely checked symptoms and often created new problems in time. Potent antimicrobial drugs further enhanced the reputation of conventional medicine. (3) The cultural effects of the Industrial Revolution. Homeopathic medicine is impossible to practice successfully in the medical "assembly line" so common in the doctors' offices of this century. (4) Infighting among homeopaths. Several severe doctrinal and political splits impaired the homeopathic community's ability to respond to the challenges of conventional medicine and cultural transitions.

The long period of declining interest in homeopathy and of attrition in the ranks of practitioners ended in the early 1970s in the United States. A sharp resurgence of homeopathic activity began then, and homeopathy has continued to grow since.

As of 1984, conservative estimates indicate there are about 1,000 medical doctors and osteopathic physicians actively involved in homeopathic practices in the United States. An equal number of other licensed health professionals—nurses, physician's assistants, dentists, veterinarians, chiropractors, naturopaths, psychologists—are also practicing homeopathy independently or with a physician. And there are an undetermined number of lay practitioners.

Homeopathy's current popularity is greatest in other countries. There are homeopaths in practically every country in the world, and homeopathy is particularly popular in India, England, France, the USSR, Mexico, Brazil, and Argentina.

In India there are over 70,000 registered homeopathic practitioners, and it is nearly as widely practiced in Pakistan. Homeopathy is well-known throughout the United Kingdom, and its practice has been growing significantly in the last ten years. The royal family has been under homeopathic care since the 1930s, and the queen is the patron of the Royal London Homoeopathic Hospital and the British Homoeopathic Association. In France over 6,000 physicians actively practice homeopathy. Over 18,000 pharmacies sell homeopathic medicines, and approximately sixteen percent of the French population occasionally or regularly use homeopathy.

There are approximately 300 homeopathic physicians in the USSR, with homeopathic medical institutions in many Soviet cities. The Central Homeopathic Polyclinic in Moscow has approximately 68 full-time homeopathic physicians and many specialty departments. Resources have informed us that there is often a two-month waiting list for appointments.

Homeopathy is readily available in most Latin American countries. In Brazil the government requires schools of pharmacy to teach homeopathy, and at least four medical schools offer classes as part of their regular curriculum. There are two medical schools offering complete homeopathic curricula in Mexico.

Understanding the basic principles of homeopathy we've presented in this chapter prepares you for "taking a case," that is, observing and recording information to help you prescribe the appropriate remedy.

CHAPTER 2

Homeopathy in Practice

THERE ARE five basic steps you'll follow when putting homeopathy into practice at home:

1. Casetaking: collecting complete and accurate information about the illness
2. Case analysis: evaluating the information you've gathered
3. Selecting the homeopathic medicine that best suits the person and his or her illness
4. Administering the remedy
5. Observing the reaction to the treatment and deciding whether to repeat or change the medicine.

Before you even begin this process, you must be able to recognize situations that are beyond your level of skill. More and more people are becoming well educated about medicine and health, and you can certainly learn to decide whether an illness can be treated at home or consultation with your health professional is necessary. The "Beyond Home Care" section included with each of the various illnesses and conditions in part 2 describes symptoms that require immediate or timely consultation with your practitioner. There are also many books covering conventional home medical care. Perhaps the most helpful are *Taking Care of Yourself,* by James Fries and Donald Vickery, and *Taking Care of Your Child,* by Robert Pantell, James Fries, and Donald Vickery. These books contain concise descriptions of all the common injuries and illnesses people encounter, along with clear instructions for determining whether home treatment is safe and how soon to see a professional.

If you do require a visit to your health care provider, he or she may still decide that the illness is not serious enough to require conventional therapies. You can then go ahead and use homeopathic treatment.

Casetaking

In preparation for casetaking it is a good idea to keep a home medical record for each member of the family. This could include pregnancy and birth history, a record of immunizations and serious illnesses or injuries, and a description of any allergies or other reactions to foods, medications, or environmental factors. You might want to jot down what you consider possible reasons for the illnesses' onset as well as comments about their severity and duration and so on.

Should you choose homeopathy to treat a particular illness, we strongly recommend you *write down* your findings as you assemble the homeopathic case. The record will ensure completeness and accuracy, and you'll have the whole case available to study at a glance. Keeping this record may also prove helpful if a similar illness occurs later, for you'll want to know how effective your earlier prescriptions were. An example of such a case record is given in the section, "A Sample Casetaking" later in this chapter.

Since homeopathic medicines are chosen to match the symptoms the sick person experiences, successful homeopathic prescription requires an accurate description of the symptoms. The homeopathic definition of a "symptom" is broader than the strict medical use of this term. For our purposes it means any change that is experienced or observed during the course of an illness. Symptoms of pain (sore throat, headache, or stomachache), physical changes (fever, flushed skin, runny nose, or skin eruptions), unusual reactions to environmental conditions or food; and the predominant emotional and mental state during the illness are all important homeopathic symptoms. Each symptom must be described in as much detail as possible to better understand that individual's unique state of psychophysiological balance.

In order to recognize the important symptoms for your casetaking, you should be aware of the homeopaths' distinctions between symptoms. For instance, "particular symptoms" are distinguished from "general symptoms." Particular symptoms refer to local symptoms associated with a specific part of the body (for example, burning pain in the throat, cold feet, throbbing pain in the back of the head). General symptoms are those felt by the entire body (exhaustion, coldness of the whole body, restlessness). Emotional and mental characteristics are considered general symptoms too, since they are felt and experienced by one's entire being. General symptoms are usually more valuable in choosing the correct medicine, since these symptoms represent the reaction of the whole body to some type of stress and, as such, represent a deeper response of the organism in its effort to reestablish health.

Homeopaths also make note of "peculiar symptoms"—that is, symptoms that do not occur in most people with a similar illness or that are simply unusual. Such idiosyncracies are sometimes even more valuable in individualizing the choice of medicine.

The method you ultimately use for taking the case will vary, depending on whether you treat yourself, another adult, or a child. If you are treating yourself, you need only run through the steps of the casetaking process outlined in this chapter. Treating others requires careful observation in addition to thoughtful questions.

Casetaking begins with a general exploration of the illness and its most obvious symptoms. Next, find out if there are symptoms affecting any other parts of the body and solicit details about how the person as a whole is reacting to the condition. As much as possible, use *the patient's own words* to record the symptoms in the outline format we show in "A Sample Casetaking" later in the chapter. Assemble a complete description of the overall illness and its separate symptoms as follows:

Contributing Causes: First, decide whether there is any apparent cause for the illness or the particular symptom. Possible stresses that made the individual susceptible to illness (other than exposure to someone who was sick) include loss of sleep, dietary indiscretions, exposure to adverse weather, or emotional stress. You may discover that a particular symptom has resulted from a different cause than the illness as a whole. For instance, after staying up late one too many nights, a person might come down with a cold and then develop a cough only because she went out in the rain a few days later.

Onset: Describe the onset of the illness and the individual symptoms. How rapidly did the symptoms develop, and how quickly do they come and go? In what order did the symptoms appear?

Character of Symptoms: Try to describe the sensations that are felt in as much detail as possible. You want to know whether the pain feels sharp, dull, bruising, cutting, burning or is of some other type. Sensations like tingling, numbness, and so forth should also be noted.

Location of Particular Symptoms: Write down the location of the pain, discomfort, or physical symptom. Be precise. Often, for example, an inflamed throat is sore on only one side, and many ear infections involve only one ear.

Modalities of Symptoms: Describe any factors that aggravate or improve each symptom. These descriptions are essential to an adequate homeopathic casetaking. You must find out what makes each symptom better or worse. These factors are called the "modalities" of the symptom, in homeopathic terminology. The more definite the positive or negative effect on the symptom, the more valuable the modality is in the choice of the remedy. It is not unusual to find that the modalities of a symptom are the opposite of what you expected. For instance, a sore throat may be improved by swallowing, and a person with a fever may feel better in a warm room. Also, the factors that aggravate one symptom may improve another, so be sure you get the specific details right. We have found from experience that almost anything may turn out to make a symptom better or worse in a particular case. See the accompanying "Outline for Casetaking in Acute Care" for a list of possible modalities to look for while casetaking.

General Symptoms: Once you've gathered information about each individual symptom, find out how the person has been generally affected by the illness. In many cases the initial investigation of the most prominent symptoms already touched upon general symptoms such as fever, energy level, and so on. General symptoms you'll want to know about include overall energy, general response to temperature, change in thirst or appetite (unusual craving or distaste for particular foods or drinks), perspiration level, change in sleep pattern, and change in emotional and mental state during the illness. The distinct modalities of each general symptom should be noted. Again, for an exhaustive list of possible general symptoms, see "Outline for Casetaking in Acute Care."

Casetaking Hints

You may be your most difficult patient. Acute illness can make it hard to concentrate, and it is hard to be objective about oneself even when well. If there is no one else in the family able to treat you, though, go ahead with the treatment process on your own.

When you take the case of another person, let the patient describe his symptoms in his own way. Limit most of your questions to the likes of "What else?" or "Tell me more about that." It is best to keep him talking without putting words in his mouth. Should he run out of things to say on his own, begin asking more specific questions about each of the symptoms, as outlined above. Make your questions as open-ended as possible, and try especially to phrase them well, to avoid yes-or-no answers. For instance, asking "How does your throat feel?" or "What makes it worse?" is preferable to saying "Does it hurt when you swallow?" or "Is it worse in the morning?" If the patient can't think of what makes a symptom better or worse, try offering a group of alternatives ("Is your cough affected by exertion, by time of day, by warm or cold air, or by position?"); or ask about a specific modality in an open-ended way ("How is your headache affected by moving around?"). If he's having trouble describing a particular sensation, give examples ("Does it feel like a pounding hammer, like an electric shock, or like a vise?").

Try to get a sense of how reliable and definite the ailing person's statements really are. You'll want to be sure of his symptoms before you use them to choose the correct medicine.

Sick people, and particularly children, may not be able to give you exact descriptions of their symptoms. Your own careful observations are meant to supplement the verbal information you collect, but sometimes they are your only source. You should note the person's *appearance*. Does she look pale or flushed; are her pupils dilated or constricted; do her eyes look puffy or heavy? Her actions should give you clues about the nature of her discomfort. She may be protecting one part of her body by covering it or by adopting a particular position. She may cry when she swallows or urinates, or she may rub or tug at her ears. Watch closely to determine the modalities of the symptoms. Observe whether factors such as time of day, temperature or weather, food or drink, or motion make the symptoms better or worse. How has the sick person's *behavior* changed? Is she more irritable, restless, sleepy, or weepy than usual? Your familiarity with her normal personality should make it easy to discern the emotional changes that accompany the illness.

Outline for Casetaking in Acute Care*

The following information should be obtained in acute care:

- Possible factors that may have led to the illness.
- Description of the onset of the illness.

Particular Symptoms:

Character of pain or any sensation (dull, aching, pulsating, pressing, shooting, numb, tingling, etc.); location, extension, and radiation of the pain or sensation.

Patterns of symptoms that occur at regular intervals or that alternate with one another.

Description (color, thickness, odor) of any discharge from the body; changes in urine or stool.

Factors that make each symptom better or worse (modalities):

Time: hour; day or night; morning, afternoon, or evening; before or after midnight.

Temperature and weather: wet, dry, cold, or hot weather; weather changes; storms or thunderstorms (before, during, or after); sun, wind, fog, or snow; open air, warm rooms, changes from one room to another, stuffy or crowded places, drafts, warmth of bed, heat of stove, uncovering.

Bathing: hot, cold, or sea bathing.

Rest or motion: slow or rapid; ascending or descending; while turning in bed, exerting oneself, or walking; upon first motion,

---

*Adapted from *A Brief Study Course in Homeopathy*, Elizabeth Wright Hubbard, St. Louis: Formur, 1977.

after moving awhile, while moving, after moving, during passive motion in a car or boat.

Position: standing; sitting with knees crossed, rising from sitting, stooping; lying on painful side, back, right or left side, abdomen, lying with head high or low, rising from lying; leaning head back, forward, sideways; closing or opening eyes; any unusual position such as knees against chest.

External stimuli: touch (hard or light), pressure, rubbing, construction (clothing, etc.), jarring, riding, light, noise, conversation, odors.

Eating or drinking: symptoms that occur during or after eating something hot or cold; swallowing solids or liquids, empty swallowing after eating any particular food; eating in general.

Sleep: before or during sleep, during first part of sleep, on waking.

Urination or defecation: before, during, or after.

Sweat or other discharges: during or after.

Coition, continence, masturbation.

Emotions: symptoms that appear or are made better or worse because of psychological states such as anger, grief, mortification, fear, shock, consolation, apprehension of crowds, anticipation, or suppression of these emotions.

General Physical Symptoms:

Strength and energy level: exhaustion, sleepiness, muscular weakness, disinclination to move; increased energy, restlessness.

Temperature reactions: effects of exposure to heat or cold, hot or cold air, other warm or cold environments, damp or dry air, or changes of temperature.

Sleep: ability to fall asleep and stay asleep, degree to which sleep is refreshing, feelings upon waking, sleeping position.

Thirst and appetite: intensity of thirst and strong preferences for hot, cold, or iced liquids; food cravings and aversions (not just likes or dislikes but actually what the person craves or hates);

appetite; food aggravations (any foods that cause general symptoms). (Note: a craving for sweets in children is not considered a symptom unless it is unusually strong.)

Sweat: its odor; when it occurs; where it occurs—on covered or uncovered parts of the body, etc.

How do the modalities listed under particular symptoms affect each of these general symptoms?

General Psychological Symptoms:

Describe all marked mental and emotional states just prior to and during the illness: feaful, anxious, sad, weeping, timid, hurried, irritable, jealous, moody, impatient, quarrelsome, obstinant, restless, obsessive, absent-minded, confused, dull, anguished, lacking confidence or exhibiting bravado, impulsive, indecisive, taking offense easily, easily startled, excitable, highly critical, lazy, malicious.

It is also important to know:

- Does the person want to be alone or in the company of others?
- Does the person like or dislike sympathy?
- How is the person affected by noise, music, or being touched?
- Is the person unusually messy or tidy?

Be sure to get as specific information as possible. For example, if the person has fears, what is he or she fearful of?: being alone, being in crowds, darkness, night, animals, illness, robbers, heights, the future, death, or whatever.

Case Analysis and Remedy Choice

Complete and accurate casetaking is crucial to successful homeopathy, but evaluation and interpretation of the symptoms you collect is probably the most challenging part of homeopathic practice. Once you've completed an accurate analysis, choosing the correct medicine is fairly simple, for you'll have a clear and reliable picture of the person's overall physical, emotional, and mental symptoms.

Finding one medicine that fits each and every symptom is usually impossible. Fortunately, this is not necessary to use homeopathy successfully. The symptoms listed were compiled from all the provings and those observed in many people. In essence, you attempt to match the symptoms to the medicine rather than the medicine to the person. In this process you first evaluate the key symptoms of the person and then assess the total symptom picture.

Case analysis consists of understanding the illness by determining which symptoms are most serious from a homeopathic perspective. Rather than focusing all your attention on a runny nose, a bad cough, or even a high fever, the important question to ask is: Which symptoms are most limiting to the person's optimal physical and psychological functioning? Sometimes a sick person feels fine generally, and only an irritated, congested nose causes him distress. But other times that runny nose is just the most obvious symptom, not the most important one—exhaustion or irritability may be causing much more misery than the sniffles.

A more analytical and mechanical step-by-step method will help you make sense of the formidable amount of information you've probably collected during casetaking. It will also help you avoid the mistake of trying to find medicines for individual symptoms or of simply picking the medicine that matches the most symptoms. As your familiarity with homeopathy grows, you'll be able to dispense with the formal analysis, as long as you remember the guidelines for symptom evaluation and case analysis. Use the following steps for case analysis:

1. *Evaluate intensity of symptoms.* The simplest test to use when evaluating the symptoms is to rank their intensity or strength. What are the most definite changes the person is experiencing with this illness? How strongly does each symptom affect the patient?

One way to gauge intensity is to consider how easy it was for you to recognize each symptom. If you're treating a family member, did the person complain to you about the problem (verbally or nonverbally), or did you have to ask what was wrong and observe him or her closely? Of course, these judgments depend on how expressive the sick person is and whether the illness has weakened him enough to limit clear communication.

Another way to evaluate symptom intensity is to ask yourself how much each symptom limits normal function. If the function of the affected system seems all right, the symptom cannot be very intense. Of course, direct statements from the individual or your own observations greatly help determine which symptoms are the strongest, most definite, or simply the worst.

We suggest you rank the intensity of each symptom on a scale of 1 to 3, using 1 to describe apparently genuine symptoms about which you're not certain or that don't seem to bother the person much, and 3 to describe intense or glaringly obvious symptoms. A commonly used method for indicating ranks is underlining the recorded symptoms one to three times, but feel free to use any method you prefer.

2. *Evaluate depth of symptoms.* Once you have evaluated the intensity of each symptom, you must next determine its "depth" or "level." As we pointed out earlier, the homeopathic understanding is that more general symptoms of the body or symptoms that affect the organs crucial to survival are the most significant manifestations of the disease imbalance. *Assuming equal intensity,* symptoms are ranked by depth from deepest to most superficial.

- Mental and emotional symptoms of deviations from the norm rank as 3.
- Physical general symptoms, including the person's energy level, sleep, fever, perspiration, thirst, and appetite, along with the effects of time, temperature, and other factors in general well-being, rank as 2. Factors associated with the onset of an illness, if definite, should be considered important general symptoms. The pace of the illness is also included in this category. Symptoms that are similar in character and that occur in different localized parts of the body may be grouped together and considered a general symptom. For example, burning pains occurring in the throat, stomach, and rectum during a digestive illness are considered one general symptom, "burning pain." The widespread muscle aches that accompany fever or the flu can also be considered a general symptom, since the aches affect the whole person (refer to the preceding "Outline for Casetaking in Acute

Care" for a more detailed listing of general physical symptoms);
• Particular symptoms, such as runny nose, nausea, diarrhea, throat pain, or other localized discomforts, should be given a 1.

Within each category rank the symptoms according to level. These judgments don't have to be exact, but use the chart of symptom levels presented in the section "Hering's Law of Cure" in chapter 1 to help you decide where each symptom fits. Among the particular symptoms, those involving the lungs, kidney, and liver are of greater importance than those of other less vital internal organs, which in turn, are more important than those of the muscles, joints, nose, and throat. Particular skin symptoms are of the least importance.

3. *Total points given each symptom for both intensity and depth categories.* List them in order of decreasing point totals for both rankings.

4. *Note idiosyncratic symptoms.* Mark symptoms on the list that you consider peculiar or unexpected. Unusual symptoms might include contradictory states, such as lack of thirst in spite of a high fever, vomiting that seems improved by eating, or a sensation of burning that is relieved by application of heat. Symptoms that aren't normally a part of a common illness pattern are included too. Of course, you may not have enough medical background to know with certainty when a symptom is atypical of the illness, but anything that seems to fit this description should be noted.

5. *Evaluate modalities.* Once your symptom list is complete, add the modalities beside each symptom. Again, rate each modality according to how strongly it affects the symptom for better or worse on a scale of 1 to 3. Modalities do not require a ranking for level, since they are only evaluated in relation to symptoms of known level. By convention, homeopaths use the symbols ">" to indicate "made better by" and "<" to indicate "made worse by" in a summary list of symptoms.

6. *List "key symptoms" of the case.* From the list you've made, select four or five symptoms of highest rank and any pronounced, unusual symptoms. Note the one or two most definite modalities of each of these symptoms. This list of key symptoms will be used to begin the process of medicine selection.

Case analysis is now complete. Collect your original casetaking notes and the list of key symptoms, and you're ready to choose the medicine.

Selecting the Right Medicine

Choosing the right medicine is essentially a matching process; you match the symptoms the sick person has with those that the medicine is known to cause in healthy people. The information we provide in this book is not as detailed as that in the reference *materia medicas* for professionals, but the main symptoms of the most commonly used medicines are listed. Each clinical chapter contains the pertinent symptoms of the homeopathic medicines most commonly used for people with that condition. The general symptoms of each medicine, along with other symptoms, are described in the *materia medica* in part 3.

The process of choosing a medicine can also be broken down into a number of steps:

1. *Read the appropriate clinical chapter(s).* If there are several symptoms (a cough and a sore throat, for example), read all pertinent chapters. Try first to match the key symptoms you listed during case analysis. Find all the medicines that fit at least one or two of these symptoms. Then read the *materia medica* descriptions of any medicine that matches the key symptoms for more details on the medicine.

2. *Make a table.* Keep track of your progress by listing key symptoms and possible remedies in a table. Check off the appropriate column for every symptom matched by the medicine being considered (see the example in the section, "A Sample Casetaking"). When you've finished the table, it will be easy to find the two or three medicines that cover the greatest number of key symptoms.

3. *Study the totality of symptoms.* At this point you should go back to the original complete case and compare *all* the symptoms with those of the medicines still under consideration. The process of selecting the right medicine requires more than mechanical matching. Subjective and even intuitive judgments can be decisive,

especially as your experience grows. The key symptoms of the case are still the most important, but you may now find that some aspect of one of the medicines just doesn't describe the remaining symptoms particularly well. Note these impressions in the table you made earlier.

4. *Choose the medicine.* Be flexible in making your final choice. Try to find a medicine that stands out as a nearly perfect match, or at least one that fits most of the key symptoms and seems to cover the overall picture. At this point, you'll have to dispense with numerical rankings and rely on reading the descriptions carefully.

As we have said, the medicine you choose does not have to cover every symptom. If, however, it has symptoms that are contradictory to key symptoms you should consider other choices. For example, people who need *Pulsatilla* are usually gentle, mild, and yielding individuals. A child who is willful and stubborn and who throws angry temper tantrums would almost never be given *Pulsatilla,* even if she had other typical symptoms that medicine covers.

Finally, if you feel that two or more medicines fit the key symptoms equally well, or that none fits them particularly well, you may have to rely less on the key symptoms and more on matching the greatest number of symptoms from the complete case. Use this method only after you've tried the other approaches.

Administering the Medicine

For the home prescriber, we recommend the use of the lower potencies: 6x, 6c, 12x, 12c, 30x, or 30c. When used according to the principles we've outlined, these potencies work well in stimulating the healing process. The 30x or 30c strengths generally act more deeply and quickly than the lower potencies, but they require more precise prescriptions than the lower potencies. If you feel uncertain about your prescription, we encourage you to use the 6x, 6c, 12x, or 12c.

In the clinical chapters of this book we will occasionally recommend the use of specific potencies. If you have the medicine but not the potency recommended, do not delay giving the medicine to the ill person. Homeopaths have found that choosing the correct medicine is more critical than finding the best potency.

Homeopathic medicines are manufactured in several forms, which are generally available in all potencies. Sometimes you can obtain the liquid *dilution* of the medicinal substance. More often this liquid has been poured over sucrose pills of various sizes, from tiny "cake sprinkle" granules (#10 *pellets*) to larger spherical pills the size of buckshot or small peas (#35 pellets). Lactose is used to prepare cylindrical tablets when the medicine has been made by the trituration process described in chapter 1.

Depending on the form in which you have your homeopathic medicines, a dose consists of one drop of liquid, ten to twenty of the tiny #10 pellets, or one to three of the larger #35 pills or tablets. Medicine bottle labels often recommend somewhat larger doses, but they are not necessary. Since the medicines are already in such dilute form, their action does not depend on a large quantity of the substance being present, and the exact amount of the dose is not critical. Giving more in no way increases the strength of the body's response. The frequency of the dose's repetition is important, however, so follow the general rules below as well as the instructions in the chapter on the specific illness.

To avoid contaminating the medicine you should not touch it. Pour it from the bottle onto a clear piece of white paper or into the bottle's cap, then tip the dose directly onto or under the tongue and allow it to dissolve in the mouth. Don't give the medicine with water. The best results occur when no taste of food, drink, or other flavors, such as toothpaste, is in the mouth. As a rule of thumb, avoid eating or drinking for fifteen to twenty minutes before and after administration of the dose.

Since the beginnings of homeopathic practice, certain substances and treatments have been found to reverse, or "antidote," the action of homeopathic medicines, and this causes the person's symptoms to return. Even relatively small amounts of substances such as camphor or coffee sometimes cause this antidoting effect. We recommend that you avoid coffee and products containing camphor or related substances during the period of homeopathic treatment and for forty-eight hours after the last dose.

Camphor is found in aromatic balms and cosmetics, including

lip balms, Ben Gay, Vick's, Heet, Campho-Phenique, Tiger Balm, Noxema, Caladryl, and some lipsticks, nail polishes, and other cosmetics. Substances containing mint or menthol, or the oils of eucalyptus, rosemary, pennyroyal, or other strong-smelling herbs are also best avoided, as are mouthwashes, cough drops, and the like.

If, for some reason, you do drink coffee or have contact with camphor or the like, you should continue treatment according to the guidelines in the following section, if no obvious changes in the symptoms occur. Since these substances do not always antidote homeopathic medicines, do not assume that they have created any problems unless you personally experience them. If the symptoms had improved but suddenly returned after the antidoting, the original medicine should be repeated. If the symptoms have changed significantly, a new medicine may be necessary, so study the case carefully.

Homeopathic medicines maintain their strength indefinitely when they are handled and stored properly, but their potency may be lost if they are treated incorrectly. The following guidelines for proper care, handling, and storage of the medicines should be observed:

- Prevent medicines from exposure to sunlight or other intense light, temperatures higher than 100 degrees, or odors of camphor, mothballs, perfumes, or other strong-smelling substances. Avoid storing them where such substances are kept, even when the medicines are tightly capped.
- Keep the medicines in their original container. They should certainly not be transferred to any other bottle that has previously contained other substances.
- Be careful not to contaminate the bottle cap and try to replace it in the shortest time possible. There also should be no strong odors in the room at the time.
- Never open more than one bottle at a time in the same room. Cross-potentization may result if this precaution is not observed.
- If more than the desired number of pills are shaken out of the bottle, throw the excess away.
- If a medicine does become accidentally contaminated, simply replace it.

Repeating and Changing the Medicine

How often you repeat the dose is crucial to effective homeopathic home care. The fundamental rule in classical homeopathy is *give no more medicine until the previous dose has ceased to act,* no matter how long or short a time that may take. Therefore no hard-and-fast schedule exists for dose repetition (ignore the recommendations printed on bottle labels); close observation of the response to treatment is the best way to tell when to repeat the medicine.

Often the person treated begins to improve markedly right after the first dose of the medicine or within an hour or two, and from there he continues to get better. Further treatment is unnecessary in these cases. Other times, however, the patient seems to pick up after the remedy is given, or a key symptom becomes less intense, and then no further improvement can be observed, and the condition gets worse again. This is an indication that repetition of the medicine is needed. You certainly should not wait until the symptoms are as bad as they were before the treatment to begin repetition.

Such close observation can be difficult. Moreover, the symptoms of acute illnesses tend to vary in the course of a few hours even without treatment. It therefore may be hard to decide exactly when to repeat the medicine. If improvement is dramatic you should stop giving the medicine. If it's not dramatic, you may give it on a flexible schedule. Each chapter on individual disease contains our recommended schedule of dose repetition for patients with that condition. In general, follow these guidelines:

1. *The more severe the person's acute symptoms, the more often should the medicine be repeated.* If the person suffers from very high fever, extremely intense pain, or other significant symptoms, or if the person is severely ill and life is threatened, medicines can be given as often as every ten to fifteen minutes (of course, in these situations obtaining medical care should be your first priority and you should only use homeopathic medicines while en route to emergency care or with the permission of your health practitioner). As the person's symptoms diminish in intensity, reduce the frequency of dosage to every one to four hours.

For illnesses that are less extreme but still have intense symptoms—high fever, bad cough, severely painful throat—you can give the medicine every three to six hours. For even less severe illnesses, such as skin problems and run-of-the-mill colds or flus, two or three doses a day are all that's usually necessary.

2. *Continue the medicine for no more than two or three days.* This should suffice if the correct medicine has been chosen. If the medicine helped at first but the symptoms returned after the first two days, you'd probably need to find another medicine.

3. *Allow enough time for the medicine to act before changing to a new remedy.* There is sometimes a delayed response, so you should give the medicine according to the schedule recommended in the relevant clinical chapter for at least twelve to twenty-four hours.

4. *Don't try too many medicines for any one illness.* Do your best to find the right medicine but stop after you've tried two or three different remedies without success.

A Sample Casetaking

Now we can apply the steps of the homeopathic method to a hypothetical case. The case will first be presented as one person would tell it to another and then in the outline form you would actually use while taking the case.

Our patient is eighteen-year-old Craig. Yesterday he came down with a sore throat that developed gradually. When he first woke up, he noticed his throat was scratchy. None of his friends or family members had been ill, and he hadn't been out in the cold. By yesterday evening he was beginning to feel quite sick with a fever of over 102°. Now he describes the sore throat as a raw, burning pain. It became much worse as the fever increased. The pain had grown somewhat worse during the night, especially on the right side. Swallowing and talking aggravate it the most, although his throat feels better for a short time when he swallows warm liquids.

Craig is also having some trouble with diarrhea. He has had two or three very liquid stools over the past twenty-four hours and has felt weaker each time, but he doesn't feel any extreme urge to move his bowels, and there is no pain.

In general, our patient's fever makes him chilly. In spite of his high temperature, he needs to bundle up with lots of blankets and can't stand a draft or cold air. He feels agitated, internally restless, and notices that his left foot is constantly tapping and wiggling. Despite the restlessness, he is so weary he can't get out of bed. He experiences some body aches, but mainly he's just very tired and sick. All these general symptoms were worse during the night, and he perspired heavily some time after midnight, after he was fully awake this morning, and he's still sweating lightly. He is about as thirsty as he normally is.

Craig feels unusually anxious, though he doesn't want to show it. He is worried that his illness might get worse, and when he woke up during the night, he couldn't help thinking that he might have a deadly disease. The anxiety and restlessness he experiences make it difficult for him to concentrate while reading his favorite magazine. He doesn't really care whether anyone else is around today, but during the night he got up and looked in on his parents to make sure they would be there if he suddenly got worse. He doesn't particularly seek sympathy, but when his mother comes in to see how he's doing, he doesn't mind her attention. Ordinarily, he leaves his records in a jumbled pile by the stereo. But earlier today when he felt a little better, he just had to get up and put them away in alphabetical order.

When he looks in the mirror he sees a pale, tired face. His throat is bright red, and there are a few tiny white spots on the right tonsil. He notices that some of the lymph nodes in his neck are a bit swollen.

That completes our description of Craig's case. The outline format you'll actually use when writing down the symptoms as you take the case will be organized in sections divided into parts of the body and the general and mental symptoms. Though you will want to be brief as you make note of the symptoms, you should write down the symptoms in the patient's own words. The case outline allows you to see all the symptoms at a glance. It's much easier to indicate the intensity of a symptom or modality by underlining and to make further notes if necessary. Here's how the case outline might look:

Main Concern: sore throat and fever since yesterday morning

Throat: had scratchy feeling in throat on waking yesterday, got worse in the evening when his fever went up now intense <u>burning</u> raw pain—

worse on <u>right side</u>, at night, <u>swallowing</u>, speaking

better from warm drinks (a little while)

Digestion: diarrhea—liquid stools two or three times only since yesterday

no pain, no urging between movements

General: <u>chilly, worse drafts of air, cold air—wants to bundle up felt sicker during the night</u>

<u>restless</u>, left foot keeps tapping and wiggling; person has difficulty reading—with the restlessness he is very tired and has to lie still in bed

no apparent reason for onset—no exposure to cold, has been sleeping and eating well

Mind: <u>anxious, worried that the disease will get worse—during the night was scared of having a deadly disease</u>

doesn't especially want company now, but during the night had to make sure that parents were there "in case"

put away records that are usually lying around in piles

indifferent to company and sympathy today

Examination: temperature is 102.5°, face pale

throat red and swollen with white spots on right tonsil

Let's try to make sense of all this information from the homeopathic perspective. Much of the work has already been done by this point if you've followed the pattern of the sample chart.

Now, with the help of the underlining you did while taking the case use the method we described in the section on case analysis, rate the symptoms of the mind, the general symptoms, and the individual physical symptoms by intensity and depth. A reminder: each symptom is rated 1–3 on the basis of intensity; for ranking the depth, symptoms of the mind earn 3 points, general symptoms 2, and particular physical symptoms 1 point. Add these two evaluations together to determine the overall rank of each symptom. Modalities are rated only according to how definite or intense they

		Rating (intensity/depth = total)
Throat:	burning sore throat	3/1 = 4
	worse on right side	2
	worse swallowing	3
	worse talking	3
	better warm drinks	2
	worse at night	1
Digestion:	diarrhea	1/1 = 2
General:	chilly	3/2 = 5
	worse at night	2/2 = 4
	restless	3/2 = 5
Mind:	anxious, worried about the illness	3/3 = 6
	more tidy than usual	1/3 = 4
Examination:	red tonsils with small white dots	1/1 = 2

Figure 2–1

are and are grouped with the symptom they pertain to. Going back over the sample chart, we can add the ratings of each symptom to the outline (figure 2–1).

Now we reorganize the symptoms, listing them in order of their ratings (figure 2–2). Note that symptoms of equal total rating are placed in order of their level, "deepest" symptoms appearing highest on the list (we may want to alter this order later).

Remember, these numerical listings are not iron-clad, and the overall case should be referred to whenever there is doubt. Still, we are ready to choose the key symptoms that we'll use for remedy selection. In this example, the first five or six symptoms qualify for key-symptom status. All have overall ratings of 4 or more, and all except the unusual tidiness are fairly well marked.

We first compare the key symptoms to those of the remedies in chapter 8 on sore throats, also consulting the *materia medica* entries in part 3. We then make a table of the medicines and the symptoms they cover as we go.

Symptom	Rating	
Anxious, fearful	6	
Chilly	5	
Restless	5	
Tidier than usual	4	
Generally worse at night	4	
Burning sore throat	4	
worse speaking	3	⎱
worse swallowing	3	modalities
worse on right side	2	
better warm drinks	2	⎰
Spots on tonsils	2	
Diarrhea	2	

Figure 2–2

The highest-ranking symptom is anxiety and fear, and this symptom is a notable feature of four medicines: *Aconite, Arsenicum, Lycopodium,* and *Rhus tox.* General chilliness is found in symptoms of *Hepar sulph.* and three of the four medicines, but not *Lycopodium.* Marked restlessness is also characteristic of *Arsenicum, Aconite* and *Rhus tox.* Only *Arsenicum* covers the patient's unusual tidiness. All three of these medicines cover the nighttime aggravation, but only *Arsenicum* is noted for the particular after-midnight increase of symptoms. All also apply to sore throats, but burning sore-throat pain is a pronounced characteristic of *Arsenicum* only. Our new table of key symptoms now looks like this (figure 2–3).

So far *Arsenicum* is clearly the leading candidate, but *Aconite, Rhus tox.,* and *Lycopodium* all cover at least three of the key symptoms. It's time to look for confirmatory symptoms. The modalities of the throat pain should help. However, all the sore-throat medicines covered here worsen during swallowing, and none are listed for aggravation from talking. Sore throat on the right side is covered by *Lycopodium* and *Belladonna.* Relief brought by warm drinks is a symptom of *Arsenicum, Rhus tox., Hepar sulph.,* and *Lycopodium.*

	Anxious	Chilly	Restless	Tidy	Worse at night	Burning throat pain
Aconite	x	x	x		x	
Arsenicum	x	x	x	x	x	x
Hepar sulph.		x				
Lycopodium	x	x	x		x	
Rhus tox.	x	x	x		x	

Figure 2–3

Diarrhea is a minor symptom in this case, but referring to the section on diarrhea shows that, of the medicines that look most promising, only *Arsenicum* is listed as appropriate.

Now compare the overall case to the pictures of each of the possible remedies. This is usually when the choice of the correct medicine becomes more clear. *Aconite* is best given in the earliest stages of acute illnesses that suddenly bring intense anguish and fearful restlessness. Arsenicum covers conditions that have progressed a little further and that are characterized by anxiety and restlessness accompanied by a greatly weakened state. These conditions also include a desire for reassuring company and a special tendency to be concerned about tidiness. The associated pains are most often burning in character, and are relieved by warmth. Digestive symptoms, especially vomiting and diarrhea, are common. *Rhus tox.* is also suited to anxiety and restlessness, but pass when the person is moving about, a characteristic that is not listed for the other medicines. *Rhus tox.* conditions typically arise after exposure to cold and damp weather, and the symptoms improve with warmth.

Based on these comparisons, we can eliminate *Aconite.* Our patient's illness did not begin suddenly, and the inflammatory symptoms did not come on with great force. *Hepar* is for someone more irritable, and *Lycopodium* is for those less chilly and thirsty. Only *Arsenicum* and *Rhus tox.* are really in the running. While almost all the symptoms of the case are covered by both medicines, *Ar-*

senicum fits most of the details of the case better, and some of its characteristic symptoms—restlessness with weakness, burning pains, tidiness—are present. Important characteristic symptoms of *Rhus tox.* that might confirm its choice are missing.

Now we must review the original case to see if we have left anything out. One detail is interesting: the patient says he doesn't care whether he has company, but when he felt afraid during the night, he had to get up to see if his parents were there. This may in fact be evidence of the *Arsenicum* tendency to seek company for reassurance.

Based on the results of this analysis, we choose *Arsenicum* as the medicine and administer it according to the guidelines in "Administering the Medicine" and the specific instructions in chapter 8. After several hours we evaluate the case again and decide whether the medicine is helping. Our next action regarding whether or not to repeat or change the medicine will be based on the guidelines in "Repeating and Changing the Medicine." If the symptoms are essentially unchanged after giving *Arsenicum* a fair try, *Rhus tox.* will be a good medicine to try next.

Well done. The clinical chapters in the following part will mean more to you now that you've experienced your first homeopathic case.

PART
2

Home Care with Homeopathic Medicine

The discussions of individual illnesses in the following chapters include descriptions of the homeopathic medicines indicated in the vast majority of cases of the conditions we cover. You'll usually find the medicine you need among those we list. Still, there is always the chance that the specific medicine required is not included, since there are far more homeopathic remedies available than we can possibly cover in this book. As your experience with homeopathy grows, we encourage you to learn to use more complete reference books listed in part 4.

Although we do not provide a separate chapter dealing with reactions to acute emotional stress, the description of *Ignatia* in the *materia medica,* part 3, provides information about the appropriate use of that medicine in some cases of emotional stress.

Before you begin to use the specific chapters, please glance through the following listing of homeopathic remedies to be found in this book and familiarize yourself with their names and abbreviations.

Table of Medicines

An asterisk* signifies those medicines we recommend be included in your home medicine kit. The dagger† signifies second-choice medicines for your home medicine kit; depending on the health problems you and your family experience, other medicines may also be included.

Aconite (Acon.)—monkshood*
Allium cepa (Allium cepa)—onion*
Anacardium (Anac.)—marking nut

Antimonium crudum (Anti. c.)—black sulphide of antimony
Antimonium tartaricum (Anti. t.)—tartrate of antimony and potassium
Apis mellifica (Apis)—bee venom*
Arnica montana (Arnica)—mountain daisy (internal and external preparations)*
Arsenicum album (Arsenicum/Ars.)—arsenic trioxide, arsenious acid*
Belladonna (Belladonna/Bell.)—deadly nightshade*
Bellis perennis (Bellis)—English daisy
Berberis vulgaris (Berberis)—barberry
Borax (Borax)—borate of sodium
Bryonia alba (Bryonia/Bry.)—wild hops*
Calcarea carbonica (Calc. carb.)—calcium carbonate†
Calendula (Calendula)—marigold (an external preparation)*
Cantharis (Cantharis)—spanish fly*
Carbo vegetabilis (Carbo veg.)—vegetable charcoal†
Caulophyllum (Caulo.)—blue cohosh
Causticum (Caust.)—potassium hydrate
Chamomilla (Cham.)—chamomile*
Cheladonium majur (Chel.)—celandine
Chimaphilla umbellata (Chim.)—pipsissewa
China officinalis (China)—peruvian bark or cinchona
Cimicufuga racemosa (Cimic.)—black snakeroot
Colocynthis (Coloc.)—bitter cucumber†
Croton tiglium (Croton)—croton oil seed
Cuprum metallicum (Cuprum)—copper
Drosera (Drosera)—sundew
Dulcamara (Dulc.)—bitter-sweet or woody nightshade
Equisetum (Equisetum)—scouring rush
Eupatorium perfoliatum (Eup. pat.)—boneset or thoroughwort†
Euphrasia (Euphrasia)—eyebright†
Ferrum phosphoricum (Ferrum phos.)—phosphate of iron*
Gelsemium (Gels.)—yellow jasmine*
Glonoine (Glon.)—Nitroglycerine
Graphites (Graph.)—graphite†
Hepar sulphuricum (Hepar sulph.)—Hahnemann's calcium sulphide*
Hydrastis (Hydrastis)—goldenseal
Hypericum perforatum (Hypericum or *Hyper.)*—St. John's wort (internal and external preparations)*

Ignatia imara (Ign.)—St. Ignatius' bean*
Ipecacuanha (Ipec.)—ipecac-root*
Iris versicolor (Iris.)—blue flag
Kali bichromium (Kali bi.)—bichromate of potash*
Kreosotum (Kreos.)—beechwood kreosote
Lachesis (Lach.)—venom from the bushmaster snake or surucucu*
Ledum palustre (Ledum.)—marsh tea*
Lycopodium (Lyc.)—club moss*
Magnesium phosphorica (Mag. phos.)—phosphate of magnesia*
Mercurius (Merc.)—quicksilver or mercury*
Mezereum (Mez.)—spurge olive
Natrum muriaticum (Nat. mur.)—sodium chloride or salt†
Natrum sulphicum (Nat. sulph.)—salicylate of sodium
Nitric acid (Nitric acid)—nitric acid
Nux vomica (Nux)—poison-nut*
Petroleum (Pet.)—crude oil
Phosphorous (Phos.)—phosphorous*
Phytolacca (Phyto.)—pokeroot
Pilocarpinum (Pilo.)—pilocarpine
Podophyllum (Podo.)—may apple†
Pulsatilla (Puls.)—windflower*
Ranunculus bulbosus (Ran. bulb.)—buttercup
Rhus diversiloba (Rhus div.)—poison oak†
Rhus toxicodendron (Rhus tox.)—poison ivy*
Ruta gravelolens (Ruta)—rue bitterwort†
Sabadilla (Sabadilla)—cevadilla seed
Sanguinaira (Sang.)—bloodroot
Sarsaparilla (Sars.)—smilax
Sepia (Sepia)—inky juice of the cuttlefish*
Silica (Silica)—silica or flint*
Spongia tosta (Spongia)—roasted sponge†
Staphysagria (Staph.)—stavesacre†
Sulphur (Sulphur)—sulfur*
Symphytum (Symph.)—comfrey*
Tabacum (Tabacum)—tobacco
Tellurium (Tell.)—tellurium
Thuja occidentalis (Thuja)—arbor vitae or the tree of life†
Urtica urens (Urtica)—stinging nettle†
Veratrum album (Veratrum alb.)—white hellebore
Wyethia (Wyethia)—poison weed

CHAPTER 3

Fever and Influenza

Fever is not a disease, but it so commonly accompanies illnesses of so many kinds that we have covered it in a separate section in this chapter. Influenza, on the other hand, is a specific type of viral infection. We cover influenza in this chapter because fever is often one of the only symptoms of the flu. We also include a brief description of Reye's Syndrome, a rare but extremely dangerous condition associated with viral illnesses.

Fever

Fever can accompany almost every type of infection and occurs in other illnesses as well. Fever may be the only apparent symptom of an illness, especially in the early stages. If symptoms other than fever are also present, consult the chapter that covers those symptoms as well.

Fever is a beneficial phenomenon, although many people are frightened by fevers and believe the slightest elevation in temperature should be brought down immediately. Fever both serves as a valuable sign that an infection is taking place and is itself part of the body's defense against the infection. Ancient physicians and scholars, such as Hippocrates and Celsus, considered fevers as a means by which the body "cooks," separates, and eventually eliminates the disease. To increase body temperature has come to be understood, in more scientific terms, as a basic biological defense shared by all organisms that can regulate their own internal temperature (Kluger 1979, 1980; Kluger and Rothenburg 1979, 1980).

Various ways fever helps fight infection have been suggested. Simple elevation of temperature reduces the growth of or even kills some disease-causing organisms. More indirect effects of fever include enhancement of such innate immune defenses as increasing the production of interferon (a chemical that inhibits viral reproduction) and increasing white blood cell mobility and activity. Fever, indeed, is an important positive response of the body.

Fever is defined as a rise in body temperature to above 99.5°F (measured orally). Normal body temperature varies from person to person and, for each person, varies with time of day, activity level, and other factors. The traditionally normal reading of 98.6°F (37°C) is only an approximate average; your own temperature may range from a little over 96° to about 99° when you're perfectly healthy. Also, after exercising or being overdressed, an elevated temperature, ranging as high as 103° in children can occur. The body's regulatory mechanisms limit fevers to a maximum of 105°–106° during simple acute illnesses in normal individuals. Higher temperatures can be harmful but, unless there is something else complicating the acute illness, a fever rarely gets so high it threatens health. Dehydration that results from fever can seriously affect children's health, but it can be prevented by making certain that extra liquids are consumed (see chapter 9).

High fevers also sometimes cause seizures in children. Such "febrile seizures" usually occur while the temperature is rising rapidly and end once it has reached its peak. They are most likely to occur in boys between six and twenty-four months old. In children who are otherwise healthy, the seizure tends to affect the whole body, not just one part or one side, and to last no more than twenty minutes, usually much less. Any deviation from this pattern may indicate an underlying neurologic disorder. Although children who have seizures during a fever need to be medically evaluated, simple febrile seizures tend to happen only once or twice and cause no lasting ill effects. They are not uncommon and generally do not represent a serious health defect.

What all this means is that the fever accompanying an acute illness is not ordinarily a cause for concern. Instead of worrying about the fever, you should pay attention to the illness responsible and try to aid the healing efforts of the body. So long as it is not too high, the fever is best left to continue its work as part of the body's effort to heal.

General Home Care

Rest and plenty of fluids are still important in the care of a person with a fever. It is normal for fever to be accompanied by a diminished appetite, so don't force-feed the patient. Allow for good air circulation in the room and make certain the patient isn't heavily covered or dressed, but protect her from drafts. Clothing should be the minimum necessary to prevent chilliness. Often these steps are all that's necessary to relieve a mild fever. We don't recommend treatment with either conventional or homeopathic medicines for minor fevers.

Sometimes bringing the fever down is a worthwhile goal in itself—if the temperature is 103.5° or higher for more than an hour, if at any time it climbs above 105°, if the patient is a child who has had febrile seizures, or if the fever simply has lasted long enough to be exhausting or really uncomfortable. But remember, fever is a protective response and you should only consider suppressing a fever for the reasons just mentioned.

Sponge bathing is an effective risk-free method to bring down fevers of those with mild or moderate illnesses. Although it is a bit uncomfortable and inconvenient, when used correctly it works more quickly than and for just as long as conventional medicines. Just have the person sit in a basin or tub in waist-deep, lukewarm water (don't use alcohol). Gradually lower the water temperature by letting a little cold water run steadily into the tub. With light brisk strokes, use a wet sponge or washcloth to bathe all exposed skin including the face. Continue for twenty minutes. Then pat the largest drops of water and allow the skin to air-dry. Protect the person from drafts during and after the bath.

When fever has risen above the levels in the previous guidelines, and if the homeopathic medicines are not working rapidly enough, you may want to use acetaminophen or aspirin. But if the patient is less than six months old, you should seek your practitioner's advice. Acetaminophen and aspirin work equally well to suppress fever, but they cause some different adverse effects. Aspirin and acetaminophen can produce side effects in lower doses and has recently been implicated in causing Reye's syndrome, a rare but often fatal disease. Acetaminophen, when taken in overdose, causes serious poisoning that can produce irreversible damage. Acetaminophen is easier to give to children because it is available as a liquid. We prefer acetaminophen to aspirin if one of these drugs must be used; they should not be used together. In any case, you must be absolutely certain they are stored in a safe place so accidental poisoning cannot occur.

Homeopathic Medicines

If you decide that the illness should be treated and fever is the only obvious symptom, consult the homeopathic information in this chapter for help with choosing the right medicine. If there are other symptoms as well (sore throat, earache, and so on), consult the appropriate chapter for relevant homeopathic medicines.

A homeopathic medicine should be given every two to six hours depending on the severity of the symptoms. Generally, the ill person will recover quickly or at least after one night's rest. If there is still fever in the morning, you'll probably want to try another medicine.

Aconite and *Belladonna* should be considered during the first stages of a sudden fever. *Aconite* is chosen for conditions that arise from exposure to dry and cold air or wind, especially if the person had been perspiring during that exposure. If he had gone outside without much clothing and then came home with a fever, consider *Aconite*. As the disease progresses, *Aconite* patients become anxious, restless, and fearful. They may toss in their sleep or throw off their covers or clothes. They are mentally alert but frightened. They have dry skin, dry coughs, and dry mouths (sometimes they have unquenchable thirst for cold drinks). Their pupils are often contracted.

The classic picture of the person for whom *Belladonna* is indicated includes a red flushed face, intensely hot skin, reddened mucous membranes, and glassy eyes with dilated pupils. The skin can be so hot that another person touching it may notice the heat lingering afterward. Although *Belladonna* patients are mentally dull and may not fully comprehend what's going on around them, they may well be restless and agitated. Children may even hit, bite, or tear at things or exhibit strange behaviors such as speaking incoherently about scary or violent hallucinations. Not all people who need *Belladonna* have these extreme symptoms, however. Still, most people who need *Belladonna* have some type of nervous excitability along with acuteness of the senses. As the illness progresses, they may develop muscle twitching, which, like many of the *Belladonna* symptoms, comes and goes suddenly.

Belladonna is by far the most commonly given medicine for people with simple fever. Even if you or your child does not have all the above symptoms, you'd probably do well to give *Belladonna*, unless another medicine is clearly indicated.

For the types of fever requiring *Ferrum phos.*, see the description given in chapter 4 on colds and coughs.

The chief indication of a fever's needing *Nux vomica* is extreme chilliness that is greatly worsened by uncovering or even slightly moving the blankets. The person can't move under the covers without setting off a wave of chilliness. The fever symptoms of *Nux* patients tend to begin after overeating, overdrinking, lacking sleep, or using drugs (either conventional medical drugs or recreational drugs). The person may also have various digestive symptoms—constipation, nausea, and heaviness of the head. The symptoms are worse in the morning and in the open air.

Although *Pulsatilla* is more often used when a person clearly has symptoms of a cold or ear infection, it may be useful when fever is the only symptom. Its primary indications during a fever are the mental and general symptoms common to all those who need *Pulsatilla.* These individuals are weepy and clinging and crave affection. Their moods are changeable. They may be irritable but the irritability is more whiny than angry or strong. They are intolerant of external heat, and the fever is markedly aggravated by warm covering or warm rooms. Their symptoms often begin after they've overeaten rich or fatty foods, and the symptoms tend to get worse at night. The *Pulsatilla* patient does not get thirsty.

See "Beyond Home Care" that follows "Influenza."

Influenza

Though illnesses such as colds, digestive upsets, and the like are often called "the flu," influenza technically refers to an acute infection of the respiratory tract associated with a particular group of viruses. Essentially, the diagnosis is influenza if respiratory symptoms like runny nose or cough are accompanied by marked fever, general weakness, and muscular aching. The person with the flu looks and feels more ill than he would with just a common cold.

Though uncomfortable, influenza ordinarily lasts only three to five days. The severity of the illness varies from person to person. Viruses have the ability to mutate, so, from year to year, some strains are more virulent than others. Bacterial infections develop when the body has been weakened by its fight against a virus. Pneumonia is a particularly dangerous bacterial complication, especially in older people. Ear and sinus infections may also occur.

General Home Care

Home treatment for people with influenza is the same as for those with fevers and colds (see chapter 4). The sick person should rest, take plenty of fluids, and be kept from extremes of temperature.

Homeopathic Medicines

One of the great success stories of homeopathic medicine concerns its superb treatment of epidemic influenza during the 1917–1918 flu season. Records maintained by government medical officers at the time showed that the proportion of patients who died from the flu or its complications while under homeopathic care was substantially lower than that of those who received regular medical treatment.

To decide on a homeopathic medicine for a person with flu symptoms, review the remedies described in this chapter and also those discussed in the chapter on colds and coughs (chapter 4). Among the appropriate flu medicines covered in other chapters are *Aconite, Belladonna, Arsenicum, Pulsatilla,* and *Nux vomica.* The medicine should be given every six to eight hours for a day or two, but if there is no improvement after the first twenty-four hours, try a different remedy. Stop as soon as definite improvement begins. In many ways, the symptoms of *Gelsemium* represent the classic picture of flu. The person mainly feels tired, weak, heavy, and sick. Generally, *Gelsemium* patients want to be left alone, not because they're especially irritable, but simply because it's too much work to interact with people. They don't feel restless, and although motion is not painful, they just lie still because they're so weak. The eyelids look heavy and droopy, and the face may appear dull and lacking in expression. The *Gelsemium* flu is characterized by chills, which often run up and down the back. There often is little thirst in spite of the fever. The nose may be runny and the throat may burn. Headaches may occur, usually in the back the head and extending to the top or forehead. The most striking symptoms, however, are general weakness and tiredness.

Like *Gelsemium* patients, those who need *Bryonia* do not want to be disturbed, but the *Bryonia* patient is indeed irritable. He may not want to answer questions. He may be preoccupied with worries about his business or other ordinary affairs. Moreover, motion makes *Bryonia* patients worse, and they feel better when lying still. They are likely to have generalized muscle and joint aches that are definitely affected adversely by motion. The patient lies still because it hurts to move, not just because he's too tired. Headache is a common *Bryonia* symptom that grows worse with motion, from walking, or even from moving the eyes. Light touch, eating, stooping, and talking may also make headaches worse; applying firm pressure and lying still relieve them. *Bryonia* patients feel generally worse in warm rooms and better in the cool air. They may have an intense thirst for cold drinks. A dry, hacking, often painful cough may accompany the flu symptoms, and constipation is also typical of *Bryonia*.

People with a *Rhus tox.* influenza are extremely restless. Their muscles become stiff and achy if they lie still for any length of time. Trying to move after a period of rest causes the worst pain for a *Rhus* patient, but she feels better as long as she can limber up and move about. She may be anxious, apprehensive, irritable, or depressed. She may be unable to sleep, because it's so uncomfortable keeping still. *Rhus tox.* patients are likely to be chilly and get worse

Beyond Home Care

Get Medical Care Immediately:

- for *any* fever in a child under four months of age;
- for fever of 106° or higher (taken orally or rectally) in any age group;
- if, with any illness whether or not there is fever, there is extreme irritability, lethargy, or mental confusion; stiffness of the neck; seizures; rapid, shallow, or labored breathing; recurrent, prolonged vomiting; or simply if the person looks terribly sick.

Get Medical Care Today:

- for any fever in a child of four to six months;
- for fever of 103.5° or higher (orally) that does not respond within six hours to home care measures, including sponge bathing, homeopathic medicine, or conventional medicine. Adults and older children who feel all right in general may wait longer;
- if fever below 103.5 has lasted longer than 24 hours in children 6 to 24 months, or longer than 72 hours in older individuals. See your practitioner sooner if you have any doubts about the severity of the illness.

If other symptoms (earache, sore throat, cough, etc.) accompany the fever, be sure to consult the "Beyond Home Care" section in the chapters that cover those symptoms.

Note: The exact temperatures we refer to are somewhat arbitrary, and when deciding to seek medical advice you must always consider the severity of the person's general illness, your experience in caring for sick people, and the patient's previous history in similar illnesses.

in cold, wet weather and better in warmth and with applied heat. Exposure to damp weather or overexertion may have brought on the illness. The patients are thirsty, sometimes only for sips of water at a time. Profuse sweating, dry mouth and lips, dry sore throat, and hoarseness often accompany the general symptoms.

Severe aching and pain deep inside the bones is the most distinctive symptom of *Eupatorium perfoliatum*. There is a bruised soreness all over the body, and the bones, especially in the back, feel as though they would break. A sudden nasal discharge with sneezing and redness in the eyes may precede the onset of these aches. *Eupatorium* patients are subject to chills, especially in the morning between 7 and 9 A.M. They may have great thirst for ice-cold drinks, but the liquids may cause digestive disorders. A dry, hacking cough may shake the whole body.

Reye's Syndrome

Reye's Syndrome is a rare but often fatal disease that usually follows a viral respiratory illness such as influenza, a cold, or chicken pox. Children under 18 are most often affected, but anyone can get it. Reye's Syndrome affects the liver and brain, along with other vital organs. Symptoms include vomiting that occurs after the onset of a viral illness, irritability, and sleepiness or disorientation progressing to coma. Diarrhea or rapid, shallow breathing may occur. Fever may or may not be present. Unlike gastrointestinal infections, Reye's Syndrome causes unexpected vomiting that is remarkable because it begins some time after the initial symptoms of the viral illness. Vomiting is usually recurrent and prolonged though this is not always the case, and it may be entirely absent in young children. Reye's Syndrome is an immediate, life-or-death medical emergency.

CHAPTER 4

Colds, Coughs, and Related Conditions

The symptoms of the common cold are the body's way of responding to a viral infection of the upper respiratory tract. Nasal discharge, sneezing, coughing, and fever are the ways the body expels and "burns out" the infecting viruses. Since these symptoms are efforts of the organism to reestablish health, they should not be suppressed unless it is truly necessary. Don't cure a cold— let a cold cure you.

Medicines such as nasal sprays, cough suppressants, and fever medicines may offer temporary relief from the symptoms of a cold, but they do so by suppressing the body's own defenses. Nasal sprays and cold capsules slow down mucus production and therefore inhibit healing, since mucus serves to cleanse the tissues of the viruses and to protect them from further infection. Cough medicines suppress the body's cough reflex, which can be problematic, since coughing helps clear breathing passages. Fever is also an important defense the body has against infection, and aspirin or acetaminophen interfere with this protective response (see chapter 3 on fever). Instead of relying on these suppressive medications, support the body's efforts by respecting symptoms and by taking homeopathic medicines.

In this chapter we review the many symptoms associated with colds and coughs, and their role in the healing process. Some consider cold symptoms—like laryngitis, croup, or bronchitis— illnesses in their own right, but we see them as various ways people react to viral respiratory infections. Therefore, we describe home-care measures that support the body's own efforts to return to health rapidly. The list of homeopathic medicines useful for cold symptoms is quite long, so we provide an index of symptoms to help you find possible medicines more quickly. (Each symptom is followed by a list of the medicines we cover that fit that symptom.)

This chapter also includes separate, brief sections on sinus congestion and conjunctivitis, or "pink eye." These conditions are closely related to colds, but we cover them individually because they may require specific home-care and homeopathic treatment measures.

Colds and Coughs

The familiar symptoms of a cold, runny or stuffy nose, sneezing, and watery eyes, along with sometimes mild sore throat or earache, are familiar to everyone. If earache or sore throat is at all marked, you should consult chapters 7 and 8 in this book. Some swelling of and tenderness in the lymph nodes is common during a cold. Most people with colds feel tired and heavy, and they also may have mild fever; when weakness or fever are predominant symptoms, influenza, mononucleosis, or some other illness may be responsible. Consult chapter 6 on influenza and the section on mononucleosis in chapter 8 for advice.

A loss of appetite commonly accompanies a cold, and there is no need to eat if you are not hungry. Bowel movements may be less frequent or may be loose.

During a cold, the body reacts to viruses infecting the lower airways, including the throat, trachea, or bronchi with coughing. Whether the cough is shallow or deep, dry or loose, depends on the location and severity of the infection and on the strength of the person's healing defenses. The viruses rarely invade the lungs themselves, and although coughs tend to drag on longer than head colds, the person almost always gets well on his own with time. On the other hand, coughs are sometimes evidence of the body's response to more serious conditions such as bacterial infection, allergy, or a foreign body in the air passages.

A variety of conditions and symptoms may affect the lower respiratory passages. The most common include the following:

Croup—caused by viral infection of the larynx (voicebox) and the breathing passages of the upper chest. Croup occurs most commonly in children three months to three years old and is characterized by a cough that sounds harsh, loud, barking, and ringing. The child is often hoarse. Because of the swelling caused by the infection, the breathing passages become more narrow and the child breathes rapidly, forcefully, and noisily as air moves through the constriction.

Croup must be differentiated from epiglottitis, which can cause sudden, complete obstruction of breathing and is a medical emergency. See chapter 8 on sore throats for details. Epiglottitis is rarely accompanied by a cough, but the other symptoms can be similar to those of croup.

Laryngitis—inflammation of the larynx and upper-chest airways that accompanies viral infection. Symptoms include a harsh, dry, barking cough low in the throat and hoarseness. The breathing difficulty characteristic of croup is absent; otherwise this is a similar illness.

Bronchitis—technically, any inflammation of the bronchi, the larger breathing tubes that lead from the trachea to the lungs. Therefore, any deep, chesty cough that is not pneumonia can be considered bronchitis. The term is used loosely but usually applies to deep, lingering coughs or to those fairly severe ones accompanied by fever but not diagnosed as pneumonia.

Bronchiolitis—infection of the bronchioles, the smaller breathing tubes branching from the bronchi in the lungs. It occurs mostly in infants no older than six months, though children as old as two years may be affected. Swelling and constriction of the bronchioles make it hard for the infant to *exhale*. These babies breathe quite rapidly and with much more effort. They look sick and anxious. Though somewhat alarming, bronchiolitis is usually self-limited and can be treated at home under medical supervision.

Pneumonia—any inflammation of the lung tissues themselves that causes fluid to form in the tiny air sacs at the ends of the breathing tubes. The fluid prevents oxygen from entering the lungs and, in turn, the bloodstream. Symptoms include a bad cough, fever, and marked lethargy, and they vary with the cause and the person's health.

Pneumonia is only a descriptive term for fluid in the lungs. It may be due to many different microorganism infections, inhalation of foreign substances, or other diseases. It is a serious illness and must be diagnosed and cared for by your health practitioner.

Wheezing—high-pitched squeaking or whistling sounds heard during breathing. It is caused by air flowing through constricted breathing tubes in the chest. Narrowing of the airways may be caused by swelling of the tubes' linings during infection, accumulation of secretions in the tubes, or spasms in the muscular walls of the passages. The person who wheezes feels short of breath and usually has particular trouble exhaling. Marked wheezing most often accompanies asthma, which we cover in chapter 13 on allergies, but wheezing may also occur during any type of chest infection or when a foreign body has been inhaled.

Sometimes a cold will set off an allergic reaction in the susceptible individual, so the situation can get complicated. If a cold or cough develops after exposure to pollen, dust, animal fur, or certain foods, if colds are recurrent, or if the cough is associated with wheezing or shortness of breath, allergy is a likely cause.

General Home Care

For simple head colds and coughs our recommendations are simple and old-fashioned:

- Get plenty of rest. Enforced bed rest is not necessary, and children can be allowed to go outdoors, but the more energy used up, the less available for healilng. Psychological stress often delays healing longer than physical activity, so try to take a break from deadlines and responsibilities.
- Drink plenty of fluids. Liquids are the best expectorant for loosening mucus and helping the body to discharge it. Illness also causes increased loss of body fluids that must be replaced.
- Blow your nose and cough phlegm out of the chest regularly. Teach children to do this at an early age.
- Use a cool-mist humidifier or vaporizer if available, and if not, try a closed bathroom with a steamy shower running. Water vapor may also help liquefy sticky mucus, making it easier to expel.
- A rubber bulb syringe may help babies too young to blow their own noses. Use the syringe to gently suck mucus from the nose

and throat. Two or three drops of salt solution (one level teaspoon in a quart of water) put into the nose will loosen thick, sticky mucus for easier removal.

- Avoid overexposure to extreme cold or heat. The energy expended in adapting to temperature stress is better used for healing.
- Although vitamin C has not been clearly proven to be effective in treating the common cold, many people who have tried it say it seems to make colds less long lasting and less severe. The recommended dose during a cold is one to five grams a day. 25 mg zinc gluconate tablets dissolved in the mouth every two hours may also be tried for up to a week.
- See chapters 6 on earaches, 7 on sore throats, and 8 on digestive problems for further home care information if the cold is accompanied by any of these symptoms.

For Croup: Croup sounds frightening but it can usually be treated at home. Using a humidifier or taking the child into the bathroom and turning on the hot shower is especially important. If the steam doesn't begin to relieve the symptoms within twenty minutes, or whenever the child has severe breathing difficulty, emergency care is needed.

For Bronchiolitis: Infants should be kept as calm as possible, for they need to conserve their energy. Cuddle them gently. A humidifier may help.

For Inhalation of a Foreign Body: Inhalation of a foreign body or substance is a relatively common cause of coughing in children, especially in toddlers who are always putting everything into their mouths. For children under six years of age, inhaling a foreign body is the most common cause of accidental death in the home. Parents should be extremely cautious when supervising children to prevent this. Young children must not be given small objects to play with, and older children should be taught not to hold things in their mouths. Peanuts and other hard, smooth foods should not be given to children under four, and all children should be kept from walking, running, or playing while eating.

Inhalation of a foreign body can cause obvious symptoms like choking, difficulty breathing, and panic. However, if the object is small enough to become lodged more deeply in the chest, or if the substance inhaled is liquid or powdery, there may be no immediate sign of a problem. Unexplained coughing or wheezing that develops suddenly or without fever (fever may occur later) should alert you to the possibility that your child has inhaled a foreign object. X-rays or bronchoscopy (a direct examination of the airways through a tube) may be necessary to make the diagnosis.

Homeopathic Medicines

Colds are usually mild illnesses and don't require treatment with medicines of any kind. We suggest you treat yourself or family members with homeopathic medicines only if the cold or cough is particularly severe or lingers more than a few days. A homeopathic medicine should be given between three or four times a day, depending on the intensity of the person's symptoms. Generally, its effects will be noticed after one or two nights' rest, although it sometimes takes longer. If no changes are observed after 48 hours, you can consider taking another homeopathic medicine if another adequately fits your symptoms.

Aconite is indicated when the cold symptoms come on suddenly, often after exposure to cold weather or cold dry wind. *Aconite* is only indicated in the first twenty-four hours or so of the illness. *Aconite* patients become violently ill within a few hours, experiencing high fever, anxiety and restlessness, sensitivity to light, and thirst. Though feverish and fearful, they are not delirious. A watery runny nose may be accompanied by violent headache or bright red nosebleed. *Aconite* is also indicated during the early stages of suddenly appearing coughs, especially croup. The child may wake early in the night with a dry, choking, croupy cough and sit up in bed and grasp his throat, feeling that he is choking. He may look frightened or even panicked and may toss about with anxiety. The cough may be dry or there may be expectoration of a little watery mucus.

The colds of *Belladonna*, like those of *Aconite*, come on suddenly, and this medicine is also indicated early in the course of the illness. Symptoms include high fever, leaping pulse, and flushed but dry face. While many medicines cover flushed skin *Belladonna* is particularly suitable when fever produces bright redness (especially of the face) and intensely hot skin. The person may experience pounding or throbbing in the head, and you may be able to see pulsations of the arteries in the head and neck. As the fever first comes on, the *Belladonna* patient is likely to be agitated, excited, or even destructive, and her senses may be hyperacute, causing irritatability and sensitivity to light, noise, odors, and so on. She is mentally dull, however, and as the illness progresses she pays little conscious attention to the environment. *Belladonna* patients may be anxious but also delirious, and have fears of imaginary things. In contrast, *Aconite* patients are alert and fear death or the dark. The pupils are usually dilated and the skin is dry during a *Belladonna* fever. The nasal discharge is thin and watery. The nose feels dry and hot, and there may be much sneezing. Sometimes the discharge dries up suddenly, bringing on severe throbbing pain in the head or face. The throat often feels raw and sore and is very red, and there may be a bad earache. There may be a dry, clutching sensation in the throat or larynx that leads to painful, scraping, spasmodic coughing from the upper chest or throat. Sometimes the cough hurts so much that a child may star to cry as soon as the urge to cough is felt. The cough sounds croupy, barking, and short. It is worse at night and may wake the individual from sleep. Only a little thin mucus is coughed up.

Like *Aconite* and *Belladonna, Ferrum phos.* is useful during the early stages of respiratory illnesses. Those who need *Ferrum phos.* are less restless than *Aconite* patients and more alert than *Belladonna* patients. The skin may be flushed with fever but not so intensely hot as it is with *Belladonna* patients. They are not delirious and do take notice of everything going on around them. *Ferrum phos.* is particularly indicated when flushing of the face is confined to well-demarcated, circular patches, where the *Belladonna* face is typically more uniformly red. During the early part of an acute respiratory infection that has few unique symptoms accompanying high fever, we recommend you give *Belladonna* first and then try *Ferrum phos.* if the former has failed.

Allium cepa (raw onion) is an easy medicine to remember since we all have had experience with the symptoms it creates. With the *Allium cepa* cold there is a clear, *burning* nasal discharge that irritates the nostrils and upper lip. There is also a profuse tearing of the eyes that does not cause irritation of the skin, though the eyes themselves may be red and burning. Both of these symptoms grow worse in warm rooms, indoors, and in the evening, and both are better in open air. Those suffering from frequent sneezing also feel better in the open air. There is often a tickling in the larynx that may lead to a dry cough so painful it makes the person grasp the throat while coughing. Though there is not much fever, the patient may be quite thirsty. Mood changes are not pronounced.

Euphrasia colds include a nonirritating, watery nasal discharge and copious burning tears—the opposite of *Allium cepa*'s symptoms. The nasal discharge is worse in open air, in the morning, and while the patient is lying down. There may be a loose cough, but it is usually not too deep or severe. Large amounts of mucus formed in the upper airways may be coughed up. The cough is worse during the day and may only occur during the daytime. It is relieved at night by eating and by lying down, though lying makes the nasal symptoms worse.

Natrum mur. can be a good medicine for those with colds, but it has few distinguishing symptoms. You should consider this medicine when the most striking symptom is simply a copious nasal flow of clear to slightly whitish mucus. The discharge is thicker and stickier than water, and it may look like raw egg whites or boiled starch. The mucus may run down behind the nose and collect in the throat. There may be sneezing spells and loss of the sense of smell and taste. A symptom that can help confirm your choice of this medicine is tiny blistery eruptions around the mouth and nose that break open to form thin crusts, such as cold sores. The lips may be dry and cracked. *Natrum mur.* patients tend to be depressed and weepy, but they don't want attention and may be made worse if you try to comfort them or offer sympathy.

Nux vomica is a valuable remedy for some people with colds, particularly with illnesses brought on by exposure to cold or to cold, dry weather. The onset of the cold is not especially sudden, and it does not tend to be accompanied by the violent symptoms or early high fever of the *Aconite* cold. *Nux* corresponds well to the dry, tickling, and scraping sensations in the nose of a cold. Initially the nose is stuffy and dry, but as the cold develops, a watery, often irritating discharge begins, accompanied by frequent sneezing. Often the nose is alternately stuffed up and runny. Stuffiness predominates at night and outdoors, runniness in warm rooms and during the day. The cold symptoms in general are made worse by eating. The throat feels raw and rough, and there may be a tickling in the larynx with a teasing, dry cough that causes soreness in the chest. The cough is worse in the morning (especially upon waking), between midnight and daybreak, in cold air, after eating, or after mental work. It gets better after warm drinks. *Nux* patients tend to be chilly and can't get warm even when they pile on the covers and turn up the heat. Every little motion of the covers causes new chills,. *Nux* is appropriate for those who are oversensitive, irritable, and easily offended.

Gelsemium colds tend to come on gradually. The person may feel less energetic for two to three days while a tickling in the nose gradually increases. When the runny nose finally starts, the discharge is watery and irritating. Particularly characteristic of a *Gelsemium* illness is the great tiredness and the sensation of heaviness felt throughout the body. The illness is accompanied by chills running up and down the back and often by a headache above the nape of the neck.

Arsenicum is useful for both head colds and coughs. There is a profuse, watery nasal discharge that burns the skin. Even though the nose runs freely, it feels stopped up. There is irritation and tickling in the nose and frequent, violent sneezing that doesn't relieve the irritation. In time the nasal discharge may become thick and yellow. The nasal symptoms may be accompanied by a dull, throbbing frontal headache. *Arsenicum* is suited for various types of coughs. The cough may come from tickling in the larynx or from deep in the chest, and it may be loose or dry. It tends to be worse during the night (especially between midnight and 3 A.M.), in cold air, or when the person becomes cold, is lying, is moving, or is drinking cold liquids. The person may cough at the sight of strangers. The cough is better after something warm to drink. Often the air passages are constricted, and there may be wheezing, especially at night. There may be chest pain, often of a burning character, especially during deep breathing. *Arsenicum* patients are chilly though, and unlike *Nux* patients, they eventually feel better if the room is made warm enough. They are anxious, restless, and fearful. In spite of their weakness from the illness, they may be overly concerned with tidiness.

Kali bichromium should be considered during the later stages of a cold. This medicine suits a thick, yellow or greenish discharge that is often distinctively ropy or stringy. It may be so thick that it can barely be blown from the nose and comes out in long strings. Crusts and mucous plugs form in the nose, and the discharges may smell offensive. A thick postnasal drip is characteristic. Sinus headaches frequently accompany the cold symptoms, often with a pressing pain at the root of the nose.

Bryonia is one of the most common medicines for people with coughs. This medicine is indicated during a cold only after it has moved down into the chest. The *Bryonia* patient's cough is usually dry and spasmodic, and it is worse when he moves or breathes deeply as well as during the day, after eating or drinking, and in warm rooms. Open air or a swallow of warm water relieves the cough temporarily. The cough is often quite painful and may cause soreness in the larynx, chest, abdomen, or back. The person may need to press the hands against the head or chest to limit painful motion while coughing. Since deep breathing and moving around may also cause chest pain, the person wants to lie perfectly still on the painful part—pressure on the sore area feels good. He wants to sigh and breathe deeply, but it hurts to do so, and respirations are shallow and panting. There is usually little expectoration; what comes up may be mucous, yellow, or streaked with a little blood. The *Bryonia* patient is thirsty and may feel too warm or too cold. He is likely to look sick, tired, and heavy and to have a dusky, dark complexion. He is irritable and wants to lie still and to be left alone.

Phosphorus is another common medicine for treating people with various types of coughs. Like *Bryonia,* it is usually not used for simple head colds. The *Phosphorus* cough may be dry or loose, croupy or deep. If the person brings up phlegm, it may be of any color or consistency, from watery mucus to thick, yellow or green pus, and may be streaked with blood. Chest pain may occur, and as with *Bryonia,* the pains worsen with motion and get better with pressure (*Bryonia* is a better choice if these symptoms are the only ones you have to work with). The chest pain is worse when the patient lies on the left side. There may be a sense of tightness, constriction, or weight in the chest. Characteristically, cold or cold air, laughing, talking, and eating worsen the cough, as does lying down, especially on the left side, and the cough also may be provoked by strong odors. It may occur at any time of the day or night, less frequently from after midnight until morning. It often comes on as the person goes to sleep or may wake her from sleep. Liquids in general and cold drinks in particular aggravate the cough. The cough may be accompanied by any type of nasal discharge. *Phosphorus* is an important remedy for those with laryngitis and hoarseness, especially when the symptoms are worse in the morning or evening. *Phosphorus* patients are chilly and crave ice-cold drinks. They are more alert than *Bryonia* patients and get nervous when they're alone or in the dark. They enjoy company and reassurance.

Pulsatilla is indicated when the mucus has become thick and yellow-green. It is bland and does not burn the skin. A fluent discharge may alternate with nasal congestion. The nose tends to run in the open air and in the evening and becomes stuffed up in a warm room. *Pulsatilla* matches both dry and loose coughs. Lying down, exertion, and warm rooms worsen the cough, which is better in open air. Deep breathing may aggravate or relieve the cough. Sometimes the cough is dry at night and loose by day. It often wakes the person from sleep. Spasms of coughing may end in gagging or vomiting (*Bryonia, Arsenicum, Drosera, Kali carb., Hepar sulph., Ipecac,* and *Lachesis* all have this symptom). The mental and general symptoms may be critical in the choice of this medicine.

Spongia is probably the most important medicine for a croupy or harsh cough (*Aconite* and *Hepar sulph.* are other strong possibilities for croup). A loud, dry cough and hoarse rasping are typical of croup. Some authors have compared the sound of the *Spongia* cough to that of a saw being driven through a dry pine log. The cough may wake the *Spongia* patient from sleep often before midnight with suffocative constriction of the throat. Excitement, talking, alcoholic beverages, lying, and ice-cold drinks worsen the cough, but drinking fluids that aren't so cold and eating may bring relief. The nose may be dry and obstructed or runny, but these symptoms are less important than those of the cough.

Drosera is another medicine for people with dry, spasmodic, croupy coughs. Probably the most distinguishing feature of the cough is a truly barking or ringing sound. The larynx is inflamed and irritated, there are clutching or constricting sensations (which sometimes get better when the patient is walking), and a tickling or roughness excites the cough. Or the cough may be in the chest, sometimes even feeling as though it were coming from the abdomen. Spasms of coughing, especially after midnight, may follow one another quickly and may end in retching or vomiting. The person may have to support the chest or abdomen while coughing to reduce pain. The *Drosera* cough is also worse while the patient is lying and may come on even as soon as his head touches the pillow. It is also made worse by eating and particularly by drinking. Though for the most part the cough is dry, there may be some mucous or yellowish sputum.

The cough of *Rumex*, or yellow dock, is dry (like those of *Drosera* and *Spongia*), but the *Rumex* cough is not so croupy or barking. The cough is dry and shallow, and it is set off by tickling in the airways, particularly in the "throat pit" just above the breastbone. Breathing in cold air especially aggravates the cough, so the person may keep the covers pulled up over his head to keep the air he is breathing warm. Even the minute temperature differences from one room to the next may cause renewed coughing. Any little irregularity in air flow may also incite the cough, so he tries to keep his breathing as shallow as possible. In fact, the *Rumex* patient may not want to talk or even listen to conversation, for he fears it might break his concentration on regulating his breathing. The cough is also worse in the evening before midnight, often around 11 P.M., and when the patient is lying down. Touching the throat may also bring on the cough (as with *Lachesis*). A fluent, watery nasal discharge with much sneezing may accompany the cough.

Lachesis is characteristically indicated by short, dry, choking coughs and violent tickling in the larynx. What little phlegm there is in the chest is brought up only with great effort. Whatever the type of cough, it is likely to be made worse after falling asleep, during sleep, or right after waking up. Exposure to cold or open air, rising from a lying position, and the slightest pressure on the throat (even from clothing) may aggravate the cough. A croup patient experiences suffocative constriction of the larynx just on entering a deep sleep, or later during sleep, and he wakes with a choking and coughing spell. He may have trouble swallowing even liquids. (Anyone who has genuine difficulty with swallowing during an acute illness may have epiglottitis, and emergency care may be necessary; see the section on epiglottitis in chapter 8.) A bad sore throat may accompany the cough. The *Lachesis* patient may be unusually excitable, impulsive, talkative, and sometimes inappropriately jealous or suspicious.

Hepar sulph. is rarely used during the beginning stages of a cold or cough. *Hepar* is used for colds that may have begun with a watery runny nose but by now have developed a thick, yellow, and sometimes offensive-smelling discharge. These patients may sneeze at the slightest exposure to cold. After exposure to cold, dry air, a croupy throat cough may be present, but the cough is less dry and more rattling than that of *Aconite* or *Spongia*. There may also be much deep, wet coughing of thick, yellow phlegm. Cold air, eating cold food, and exposure to the wind worsen the *Hepar* cough. Uncovering brings on the cough to such an extent the *Hepar* patient may cough if she puts a hand or foot out of the covers. The cough is also aggravated in the evening before midnight and by deep breathing. *Hepar* patients are irritable, sensitive to touch and cold, and they feel better in warm, moist weather.

Ipecac is especially valuable in treating infants' bronchitis or bronchiolitis, although older individuals often need this medicine too. These illnesses come on fairly rapidly, spreading from a simple head cold down into the chest within a day or two. By the time the person needs *Ipecac*, the cough is deep and wet, marked by coarse, loud rattling and accumulation of much mucus in the chest. The phlegm and the spasmodic cough cause choking and suffocation, and the patient may have trouble getting her breath. Phlegm comes up with difficulty. As is typical during bronchiolitis, breathing out may be especially harder than breathing in. Spasms of nearly incessant coughing may occur, ending in retching, gagging, or vomiting. *Ipecac* should be considered even for dry coughs if gagging or vomiting are severe, whether or not the patient is nauseated. The cough is usually worse in a warm room. There may be a stuffy nose and sneezing and sometimes bright red nosebleeds. Mentally, the *Ipecac* patient may be full of desires but doesn't really know what she wants, and she may reject things she has asked for when she gets them. *Ipecac* children are often quite irritable.

Like *Ipecac*, *Antimonium tartaricum* is indicated when the person has a rattling cough and a chest full of mucus. The symptoms of this medicine come on more slowly than those of *Ipecac,* however, and *Antimonium tart.* is usually given during the later stages of a progressively worsening cough. In these cases the sputum is not difficult to raise, but the person is just too weak to cough effectively and can't clear his chest. Breathing sounds rattling, and as the mucus builds up, the patient becomes short of breath. He is quite ill and exhausted and may look drowsy and pale, sometimes with sunken features and slightly bluish skin (these symptoms require medical evaluation).

The *Rhus tox.* cold or cough symptoms usually include a congested nose with a thick, yellow or green discharge, a red and scratchy throat, and a dry cough with tickling behind the upper part of the breastbone. Hoarseness is common. The cough worsens in cold rooms or in cold, wet weather, with the slightest uncovering, during deep breathing or lying, after bathing, and in the evening or during the night. The cough may prevent sleep or come on during sleep, sometimes waking the person. Motion may make the cough better. In general, the person is restless and feels better when moving about.

A patient can develop the symptoms of *Dulcamara* during or after exposure to cold and wet weather, when wet or chilled, or when experiencing a sudden temperature change from hot to cold. If the onset of the illness is related to this kind of exposure, and if there aren't enough symptoms to indicate another medicine, you should try this one. All kinds of nose and cough symptoms are covered by this medicine. Sometimes the cold symptoms are accompanied by neck pain and stiffness from the cold damp weather.

The *Kali carbonicum* cough, whether dry or wet, is violent and spasmodic and is particularly severe in the early morning hours, between 2 to 5 A.M. Needle-like pains in the side commonly accompany the cough. The pains are worse during breathing and coughing but are not particularly aggravated by motion. They tend to be worse on the right side of the chest. The cough itself is made worse by the patient's breathing cold air, becoming cold, moving or exerting energy, and lying, especially in the evening or at night. There may be choking, retching, or vomiting along with the cough. The sputum may be difficult to bring up even though at times there is a lot of it. It may look mucous or thick and yellow. The throat may feel as though a splinter or fish bone were caught in it (also a symptom of *Hepar sulph.* and *Lachesis*). The person is usually thirsty and chilly and is often sweaty. He may be irritable and yet want company, and he is often full of fears.

Repertory for Cold and Cough Symptoms

Since there are so many medicines to consider when treating a person with a cold or cough, the following index of symptoms, or

---

Beyond Home Care

Please refer to the beyond home care section in chapter 3 on fever and influenza.

People with a common cold may be more susceptible to secondary bacterial infections like ear infections, sinusitis, strep throat, lymph node infections, and pneumonia. Check chapters 7 and 8 and the section on sinus conditions in this chapter for more information on how to treat such conditions and when medical care should be sought.

Get Medical Care Immediately:

- if something is inhaled that can't be coughed out completely, even if there isn't any obvious breathing difficulty at first. This includes inhaling powders and liquids, though small amounts of water won't generally be a problem;
- if there is severe headache, extreme weakness, convulsions, or stiffness of the neck.
- if there is marked irritability or confusion
- if there is severe breathing difficulty or chest pain.

Call Your Practitioner Immediately:

- if vomiting begins unexpectedly during the course of the illness repertory, will help you find the medicines most likely to cover the case. Compare the main cold and cough symptoms of the case to those listed in the repertory, writing down the medicines listed under each symptom. Then, to make your final choice, read the

Get Medical Care Today:

- if fever has persisted. See chapter 3 for specific advice for each age group;
- if the symptoms have been accompanied by marked weakness and have lasted longer than a week or so;
- if stools are very light in color, if urine is very dark, or if there is yellowing of skin or eyes;
- if there is breathing difficulty, shortness of breath, or much more rapid breathing than normal. Babies with any breathing difficulty must be examined. A respiratory rate of greater than 50 breaths a minutes *at rest* in young children, above 40 in children older than two, or over 30 in individuals older than ten should prompt at least a phone call to your practitioner;
- if any wheezing occurs for the first time or if there is moderate or severe wheezing at any time.
- if there is significant chest pain.

See Your Practitioner Soon:

- if mild cold symptoms have been persistent for more than three weeks.

See Your Homeopath:

- if you get recurrent colds. Everyone gets an occasional cold, and children between three to six years of age get an *average* of eight colds a year. As long as the illnesses clear up fairly quickly and aren't severe, you should not be concerned. Susceptibility to frequent or severe colds does indicate a weakness of the healing defenses, and constitutional homeopathic treatment can build strength and resistance.

written descriptions of the medicines that you've found in the index of this chapter and the *materia medica* section. Medicines printed in the repertory in all capital letters are most strongly indicated for that symptom.

REPERTORY FOR COLD AND COUGH SYMPTOMS

I. Head Colds

Early stages of a cold: ACON., BELL., FERR. P.
Most common medicines for head colds: ALLIUM, ARS., BELL., EUPHR., GELS., KALI B., NAT. M., NUX, PULS.
Nasal Discharge
   Green: Bry., KALI B., Kali C., Phos., PULS., Rhus
   Offensive: HEP., KALI B., Kali C., Lach, Phos., PULS
   Ropy or Stringy: KALI B., Phos., Spong
   Thick: ARS., Hep, KALI B., Kali C., Nat M., Phos., PULS., Rhus, Spong
   Watery: Acon, ALLIUM, ARS., Bry., EUPH., Kali B., Nat M., NUX
   White mucus: Ars., NAT M., Nux, Phos., Puls.
   Yellow: Ars, HEP, KALI B., Kali C., Lach., Nat M., Phos., PULS
Nasal Discharge Modalities
   Worse morning: Acon., Euph., NUX
   Worse night: Kali B., Rumex
   Congested at night: Nux
   Worse in open air: Dulc., Kali B., Phos., PULS.
   Better in open air: Allium, NUX, Puls.
Nasal Discharge with Chilliness: Acon., Ars., Bry., NUX, Puls., Spong
Fluent Discharge with Cough: Allium, Ars., BELL., EUPH., Ferr. P., Gels., IPEC., Kali B., Nat. M., Phos., Rhus, Spong
Fluent Discharge with Fever: Acon., Ars., Bell., BRY., Hep
Fluent Discharge with Croup: Acon., Ars., Hep, Spong
II. Coughs

Most common medicines for coughs: ACON., ANTI. T., ARS., BELL., BRY., DROS., FERR. P., HEP., IPEC., KALI C., LACH., PHOS., PULS., RHUS, RUMEX, SPONG.
Dry cough: ACON., ARS., BELL., BRY., Dros., Dulc., Ferr. P., Hep.,

Kali B., KALI C., LACH., NAT. M., NUX., PHOS., PULS., Rhus, RUMEX, SPONG
Loose cough: ANTI. T., ARS., Euph., Hep., Lach., Phos., PULS.
Croupy cough: ACON., Ars., Bell., DROS., Hep., Kali B., Lach., Rumex, SPONG
Cough Modalities:
 Worse after bathing: RHUS
 Worse from cold: ARS., Bry., Dulc., HEP., Kali B., Kali C., Lach., NUX, PHOS., RHUS, RUMEX
 Worse from cold drinks: ARS., Phos., Spong
 Worse from cold foods: Hep.
 Worse from cold wet weather: Dulc.
 Worse in the day: Bell., Bry., EUPH., Ferr. P., Kali C., LACH., PHOS.
 Worse from deep breathing: ARS., Bry., DROS., Hep., Lach., Phos.
 Worse from drinking: Ars., Bry., DROS., Hep., Lach., Phos.
 Better from drinking: Bry., SPONG.
 Better from warm drinks: ARS., BRY., NUX, RHUS, Spong.
 Worse after eating: Ant., Ars., Bry., Ferr. P., Hep. Ipec., KALI B., Kali C., NUX, RUMEX
 Worse after exertion: Kali C., Nat. M., Nux., PULS.
 Worse from laughing: Phos.
 Worse from lying on the left side: Phos., Rumex
 Worse from lying down: Ars., Bry., Dros., Dulc., Kali C., Lach., Phos., PULS., Rhus, RUMEX, Spong.
 Worse in the morning: ARS., EUPH., KALI B., KALI C., Nat. M., NUX, PHOS., PULS., RUMEX
 Worse from motion: Ars, Bry, Kali C., Nux, Phos.
 Worse at night: ACON., ARS., Bell., Dros., HEP., IPEC., KALI C., LACH., Nat. M., Phos., PULS., Rhus, Rumex, Spong.
 Worse in the open air: Acon., ARS., Hep., Lach., PHOS., Rhus, RUMEX
 Better in the open air: Allium, BRY., PULS.
 Worse from talking: Bell., DROS., Euph., Hep., Lach., Phos., RUMEX, Spong
Chest pains during cough: Acon., BELL., BRY., DROS., PHOS., PULS., RHUS, SPONG.
Throat pain during cough: Acon., ALLIUM, BELL., Bry., Hep., Kali B., Kali C., Lach., Phos., Puls., Spong.

Sinus Problems

The sinuses are cavities in the bones above the eyes and around the nose. Normally, they are filled only with air. During a cold or allergic reaction, the membranes that line the sinus cavities may swell and produce excessive mucus. If the openings from the sinuses into the nose are blocked by swelling, the pressure of the air trapped inside and the buildup of mucus cause sensations of stuffiness and fullness in the face. The nose is stuffed up. When the sinuses are involved during a simple cold but there is not bacterial infection the condition is sometimes referred to as "sinus congestion."

A true sinus infection results when bacteria enter a blocked sinus cavity and thrive and multiply in the trapped mucus fluid. Inflammation increases and pus is produced, and throbbing and pressure in the sinuses increase. If the lower sinuses are involved, the teeth hurt or feel too long. The infected sinuses make the parts of the face definitely tender to touch. A thick, yellow-green nasal discharge is produced, but it may not be that profuse because of the blockage. Fever and tiredness usually accompany the illness, and the person can become very sick.

General Home Care

Sinus congestion and mild infections can be cared for at home. Home care is simple. Rest is essential. Drink plenty of liquids, and use a humidifier to help thin and loosen the secretions.

Homeopathic Medicines

Consider the medicines listed here first when treating someone with a sinus infection. All of these remedies cover thick, yellow to green drainage from the nose. You can also consult chapter 12 on headaches and the medicines covered earlier in this chapter for colds and coughs in general. Give a dose of the medicine every eight hours or so, stopping if there is improvement. Switch to another remedy if the symptoms aren't getting better after a day.

Kali bi. is one of the most helpful medicines for people with sinus pain and congestion. It's especially indicated when pain or pressure is worst above the root of the nose and when the discharge is particularly thick, stringy, or tough. Pain may also occur in the forehead, often over one eye or shooting to the outer angle of an eye. The pain may be confined to small, particularly localized spots. The symptoms often begin in the morning, get worse by noon, and go away in the late afternoon. Cold weather, stooping, motion, and walking make them worse. Pressure, warmth, and warm drinks help relieve the pain.

Pulsatilla should be considered when the sinus pain is worse at night, in a warm room, or with standing, stooping, or raising the eyes. The pains lessen in the morning and with pressure. Digestive symptoms such as nausea or indigestion may accompany the sinus pains.

People who need *Silica* have sinus pains distinctively improved with pressure, and such people may want to keep the head wrapped up tightly. They also feel better after warm applications. Their pains are worse with cold, mental exertion, noise, motion, stooping, talking, and light touch.

Spigelia should be considered when sinus pain begins after exposure to cold or cold, wet weather, or when pain is much worse with stooping or bending the head forward. The head symptoms are relieved by cold applications or washing with cold water, and warmth is aggravating. The pains are also made worse by motion, jarring, noise, and light, whereas lying down with the head propped up improves them.

Beyond Home Care

Get Medical Care Today:

- if there is marked fever, severe pain, or foul-smelling discharge;
- if there is evidence of mild sinus infection (tenderness, thick yellow or green discharge) with no improvement after forty-eight hours.

If the pain is made much worse by cold or touch, *Hepar sulph.* is probably the remedy. *Hepar* is particularly indicated for pain concentrated at the root of the nose that is worse in the morning. The scalp and whole head may feel bruised and sensitive to touch or to simple movements of the head or eyes.

Conjunctivitis

The conjunctivae are the thin transparent linings that cover the surface of the eyes and the inner eyelids. Infection, allergy, or exposure to irritating chemicals can cause inflammation and swelling of the conjunctivae, and the affected eye tears and looks bloodshot. This condition is known as conjunctivitis, or "pink eye."

Both cold viruses and various bacteria can infect the conjunctivae. When the conjunctivae are infected with viruses, the discharge from the eye is clear and watery. Bacterial infections result in a thick, yellow-to-green discharge.

Usually the symptoms begin in one eye and spread to the other within a few days. The affected eye is bloodshot and the lids may be puffy and a bit red. The eyes may feel tired or as though sand had got in them. The eyelids often stick together as the discharge dries, especially during sleep. Vision is not affected, except by the discharge that covers the surface of the eye.

These infections are not dangerous as long as they do not move into deeper layers of the eye, an uncommon occurrence. Even without treatment they clear up within ten days or so. Conventional practitioners give antibiotic eyedrops when bacteria are thought to be responsible for the infection, but there are no effective drugs for ordinary viral conjunctivitis.

Allergic reactions and irritation from smoke, smog, or other chemicals can cause similar symptoms of redness and tearing. You can readily distinguish these conditions from infectious conjunctivitis in most cases. Generally the infectious types are accompanied by cold symptoms or occur after exposure to someone else with the infection. When the conjunctivitis is caused by allergies or chemical irritation, you can usually remember the exposure to pollens, dust, fumes, or the like that led to it. Allergies and irritation usually begin by affecting both eyes and typically cause a watery or slightly mucous discharge. Allergic conjunctivitis is the only type frequently accompanied by much itching.

General Home Care

Avoid rubbing the affected eye(s) for this can injure the inflamed, weakened tissues and drive any infection into deeper layers of the eye. Touching the eye also spreads the infecting germs to your other eye and to other people. Periodically cleanse the eye with warm water to remove discharge and crusts. Be careful not to touch the unaffected eye, and be sure to wash your hands well every time you do touch your eyes or the surrounding area. If the conjunctivitis is caused by an allergy or irritant, rinse the eyes with artificial tears, sterile normal saline solution, or over-the-counter eyedrops, all available at a pharmacy.

Homeopathic Medicines

Give a dose of the indicated remedy three or four times a day for up to three days. Stop as soon as symptoms definitely improve.

Belladonna can be given in the earliest stage of conjunctivitis, when the main symptom is sudden onset of bright red, bloodshot inflammation of the membranes. The eye feels hot and may throb. Clear tears flow copiously. Light bothers the eyes (if this symptom is at all severe, see your practitioner).

Euphrasia (Eyebright) has a well-deserved reputation, in both homeopathic and herbal traditions, for helping people with eye troubles. *Euphrasia* conjunctivitis is characterized by the copious flow of acrid, watery tears that burn the face. With time the discharge may become thick and mucous but never opaque or yellow-green. Often the eyes feel dry or as though there were dust or sand in them. The eyes and often the lids (especially the margins) are very red. There may be an accompanying nasal drainage (see "Colds and Coughs").

Apis is the medicine to use when swelling of the conjunctivae is extreme and there is marked aggravation from heat. The conjunctival lining of the inner eyelid may be so swollen that it protrudes from behind the lid. The conjunctivae on the eyeball itself may be so swollen the iris looks like it is sitting in a shallow depression (see your practitioner if swelling is this severe). The lids themselves and the areas above and below the lids may be puffy and swollen as if they were full of water. The eyes and often the lids are quite red. There are gushing, hot tears. The eyes may sting or burn, and the discomfort is worse in a warm room. Cold bathing of the eyes brings relief.

Pulsatilla may be curative for infections characterized by discharge of much thick, yellow-to-greenish matter from the eyes. The discharge generally does not irritate the skin, but the eyes may itch and burn, especially in the evening. The lids, especially the margins, may also itch intolerably. Going out in the open air as well as bathing the eyes in cold water afford relief. These eye symptoms may accompany a typical *Pulsatilla* cold, and the general symptoms of the medicine may be present.

Mercurius should also be considered when the discharge is yellow-to-green, but in this case the liquid is often irritating to the skin and may be less thick than the *Pulsatilla* discharge. Nighttime, warmth of the bed, and the glare of firelight may worsen symptoms of discharge and smarting of the eyes. There are likely to be eruptions of whiteheads or scales around the eyes and on the lids.

Consider *Hepar sulph.* if there is a thick, puslike discharge, if eye discomfort is aggravated by cold and relieved by warmth, and if the general symptoms of the medicine are present.

Blocked Tear Duct

The tear ducts at the inner corners of the eyes allow the tears, which are constantly being formed, to drain. Some newborn babies' tear ducts are too small, causing the tears to back up into the eye and nourish the growth of bacteria. The child has a constant, thick, yellow or green discharge of pus dripping from the eye. The eye itself is usually not involved and doesn't look badly bloodshot or swollen. This condition may last for a few months before the passageway of the tear duct grows.

Constitutional homeopathic treatment is generally the best way to help the child with this condition, unless the tear duct is completely absent and must be opened surgically. If you cannot obtain constitutional care from a homeopathic professional, you can try giving the child *Silica* 6x once or twice a day for ten to fourteen days. Conventional practitioners use antibiotic drops or attempt to dilate the tear duct with an instrument.

Beyond Home Care

Get Medical Care Immediately:

- for severe eye pain;
- for any loss of vision;
- if there is an injury to the eye or a foreign body or chemical in the eye.

Get Medical Care Today:

- if there is any significant eye pain;
- if light causes pain in the eye;
- if the pupil is shaped irregularly or does not react to changes in light;
- if the worst redness definitely exists in a circular pattern around the iris;
- if the area over the inner eye's tear duct is swollen or red.

Call Your Practitioner Today:

- if there is a thick, yellow or greenish, puslike discharge dripping from the eye.

CHAPTER **5**

Childhood
Illnesses

In this chapter we cover teething, bed-wetting, and the infectious illnesses commonly associated with childhood— measles, german measles, mumps, and chicken pox. Of course, adults can get these infectious diseases too, especially today, as better hygiene and immunizations have kept many grown-ups from exposure to infection in childhood. The symptoms of these illnesses are essentially the same in adulthood and childhood, although we make note of what differences there are. Our comments about childhood infectious diseases thus apply to adults as well as children.

Teething

Although the eruption of teeth through the gums is always uncomfortable, some children suffer terribly every time new teeth come in. In recent years, the treatment of teething children has probably convinced more people of the efficacy of homeopathy than anything else.

General Home Care

Rely on simple home care measures for your teething child unless symptoms are severe. Offer her something soft but firm to gnaw on. Ice wrapped in a moist washcloth or a commercial, frozen teething toy may help.

90

Homeopathic Medicines

If the child is irritable and suffers a great deal of pain in spite of your efforts, try a homeopathic medicine. Give the dose no more than three times a day and only when symptoms are severe. Stop as soon as she improves.

Chamomilla is by far the medicine most likely to help the teething child. The gums are inflamed and the child can't keep her fingers out of her mouth. One cheek may be hot and red while the other is pale. She screams with pain and nothing can comfort her. She is terribly irritable. She demands things but rejects them as soon as she gets them, tossing them across the room if she's old enough. She may throw angry fits, screaming and hitting those around her. She is calm only if she is constantly carried about or rocked. During sleep she tosses about and cries out suddenly.

Ignatia may help if the child is extremely distressed by the pain but not so irritable. She sighs, sobs, and cries. She may tremble and single parts of the body sometimes quiver or jerk. She may wake from sleep with piercing cries.

The *Kreosote* child suffers from extremely painful dentition. The gums are severely inflamed and red with a spongy consistency. The child is agitated and wakeful.

Bed-wetting (Enuresis)

Most children are ready for toilet training between the ages of two and three. Bowel control usually comes first, followed within six months or so by daytime control of the bladder. Staying dry at night is a little more difficult, though, and bed-wetting is considered normal until the child is six or so. Even after that age, while various tests may be considered, in all likelihood this problem will eventually clear up on its own.

Though it seems automatic, nighttime bladder control is still a function of the higher brain, and it just takes time to learn this neurologically complex skill. How early a child learns to control his bladder does not reflect any other aspect of his psychological or physical development, as long as there are no other symptoms. Of course, concern about persistent bed-wetting is natural, and neither child nor parent likes the wet sheets and forced clean-up routine. Try to give your child acceptance and reassurance, however. Communicating anxiety or dissatisfaction with your child does not help him learn bladder control and may actually aggravate the problem.

There can be other causes of bed-wetting. Sometimes genetics is a factor, since the tendency to wet the bed runs in families. A child's food sensitivities or allergies may also play a role. Pediatrician Lendon Smith has estimated that reactions to such foods as milk, citrus fruits, chocolate, and sugar contribute to the problem in as many as one tenth of all bed-wetting children.

Psychological factors can be responsible for bed-wetting. Stress can put demands on the child's psychological defenses, limiting the nervous system's capacity to learn new skills. Sometimes the child unconsciously uses bed-wetting as an easy way to get attention. In other cases wetting the bed may be an expression of bottled-up anger. Some children stop wetting the bed but then start again after facing a stressful situation or illness. The birth of a sibling, a move to a new home, or a serious illness may trigger the recurrence of bed-wetting.

On rare occasions infection or structural abnormality of the urinary tract is responsible for bed-wetting.

General Home Care

The primary treatment for bed-wetting is "tincture of time," allowing the child to learn to control his bladder at his own pace. Helpful factors include providing a secure, guilt-free, loving home environment. Encourage his efforts to stay dry at night, just as you would encourage his efforts to draw or to ride a bicycle. You might also try gentle suggestions that allow his subconscious mind to associate urinating with being out of bed. For instance, every time he urinates, have him say something like, "My feet are on the floor. Now I'm going to the bathroom."

Limiting fluid intake during the latter part of the day and having the child urinate just before bedtime are traditional but unsuccessful measures for controlling bed-wetting. Some parents have a little better luck getting the child up to urinate during the night, especially if he wets the bed at a predictable time.

Since food allergies may be the reason for your child's bedwetting, consider eliminating possible offenders from your child's diet and see how it affects his bed-wetting. Remember, it's often the foods the child craves most that he is sensitive to.

Constitutional homeopathic treatment can sometimes be helpful to bed wetters, but we are not tremendously impressed with the results. We have seen some children stop bed wetting immediately after receiving a constitutional medicine, but more often there has been no apparent change in this symptom, even when the child improves in other ways.

The most helpful role your health practitioner is likely to play is in reassuring you that your child is healthy. If bed-wetting persists past the age of six or so, the practitioner will want to run tests on the urinary system to rule out infection or anatomical problems. He or she will also consider the role of stress and psychological factors. If any problems are discovered in any of these areas, appropriate treatment can be given. Rarely is surgical or medicinal treatment necessary.

Some practitioners prescribe powerful drugs such as imipramine (an antidepressant), dilantin (an anticonvulsant), or detroamphetamine (an amphetamine) for bed-wetting children. We are of course against treatment that suppresses symptoms without dealing with the underlying imbalance, especially treatments involving powerful drugs with many potential adverse effects.

Homeopathic Medicines

Generally, the best way to use homeopathy to help children who wet the bed is with constitutional treatment. Seek professional homeopathic care for this treatment. If this is unavailable, you may try one of the following medicines as long as there are no other health problems. Give a single dose of the medicine and allow four weeks to pass between repetition of the medicine or before trying a new one.

Causticum is probably the most common medicine given to children who wet the bed soon after falling asleep. They tend to wet the bed more often in the winter, on cold days or nights, during changes in the weather, and less often in the summer. They may also dribble in their pants during the day while coughing or sneezing

Beyond Home Care

See Your Health Practitioner Today:

- if there are any other symptoms associated with the bed-wetting: frequent or painful urination, bloody urine, abdominal pain, or fever. Even if these symptoms are more mild, your child needs medical evaluation within a day or two.

See Your Practitioner Soon:

- if your bed-wetting child is over six years old;
- if your child has learned bladder control but has been wetting the bed again regularly for a month or so.

or after any excitement. They seem to pass the urine so easily they are unaware of the stream until they have created a puddle.

Equisetum is also commonly given to children who wet the bed. *Equisetum* is indicated, after the primary stresses that led to bed-wetting have been dealt with, when the child still wets the bed mostly out of habit. Such children may experience a dull pain in the bladder and a sense of distention that is not relieved by urinating.

Sepia is given when the child urinates shortly after going to sleep (a *Causticum* and *Kreosotum* symptom as well). It is most often prescribed for little girls who are emotionally cold and hate sympathy, who want to be alone, and who have some of the other typical *Sepia* general symptoms.

Kreosotum is indicated when the child urinates and dreams of urinating. As with *Causticum* and *Sepia,* the child usually urinates shortly after falling asleep. The child tends to sleep very deeply and often is quite difficult to awake.

Belladonna is given to bed-wetting children who sleep restlessly, moaning and perhaps even screaming in their sleep. They are difficult to awake and are usually delirious. They may also pass urine during the day, especially while standing.

Pulsatilla is the medicine of choice for sensitive, weepy and gentle children (usually girls) who wet the bed. They often sleep on the back with hands above the head or on the abdomen. They are more apt to wet the bed if the room is warm or stuffy.

Measles

Measles is one of the most contagious diseases known. It has become a rare disease in the United States, but some children still do get measles and the illness can be serious.

The symptoms of an early case of measles are identical to those of a bad cold. After an incubation period of ten to fourteen days, the symptoms begin with a hacking cough, nasal discharge, and a low-grade fever. Redness and watering of the eyes, along with sensitivity to light, are usually pronounced. After a few days, small white spots resembling salt crystals appear inside the mouth on the inner cheeks.

Within four or five days after the symptoms begin, there is a brief drop in fever, and then the classic measles rash develops as light red spots on the face and sides of the neck. The spots come out in small, irregularly shaped blotches that may be flat or slightly raised. As the rash rapidly spreads, the blotches run together, and new ones appear on the upper chest and arms. Over the next few days the rash spreads over the back, abdomen, and legs, eventually reaching the feet. By about this time the fever drops and the child starts to feel much better.

General Home Care

A child with measles usually has a diminished appetite. Don't try to force-feed him if he isn't hungry. His body is telling him that he doesn't need the food, or at least that he can't digest it efficiently. With such a high fever, he is at risk of dehydration (see chapter 9) so make sure he receives enough liquids. The child's sore and inflamed eyes are likely to be sensitive to light. Keep the lights dimmed.

Homeopathic Medicines

The homeopathic medicine you choose should be given every four to six hours for no longer than a couple of days. If you notice no changes after three days, you may consider trying another medicine. According to Samuel Hahnemann, *Aconite* is "almost miraculous" in the treatment of measles; E. A. Farrington, a nineteenth-century, American homeopathic authority, said it's "the best remedy for the beginning of measles." *Aconite* is primarily useful early in the course of the disease, especially if it has come on suddenly. At this point you won't know for certain that the illness is measles. There is fever, restlessness, nasal discharge, red eyes, photophobia, dry croupy cough, chest stitches, restless sleep, and sometimes diarrhea.

Like *Aconite*, *Belladonna* is useful during the early stages of measles, but it can also be used after the rash has erupted. *Belladonna* is particularly indicated when predominant symptoms include a red face, throbbing headache, and moistened skin from the fever. These children are drowsy and at least a little delirious but may be unable to sleep. Their limbs may twitch or jerk. Light, noise, or the slightest jarring makes their symptoms worse.

Gelsemium is a third medicine possibly useful during the early stages of measles. Unlike *Aconite* or *Belladonna*, the *Gelsemium* measles begins slowly. There is a gradual onset of fever and chilliness, and the child feels heavy and very tired. Sometimes raising the head or even keeping the eyes open is just too great an effort, and the child lies motionless. She is apathetic and doesn't want to be disturbed. The *Gelsemium* child is usually not very thirsty and is apt to have a watery discharge that burns the upper lip, a headache above the nape of the neck, and perhaps a harsh, croupy cough. *Gelsemium* may be used during the rash stage of measles as well.

A prescription of *Euphrasia* is indicated during measles when the nasal discharge and the eye symptoms predominate. As distinct from that of *Gelsemium*, the *Euphrasia* type of nasal discharge is profuse and does not burn the upper lip. These children do, however, have acrid tears that stream out of their eyes. The eyes appear red or unusually bright. Sensitivity to light is especially intense.

Their nasal and eye symptoms tend to improve in the open air. They have a dry cough and possibly hoarseness. They also tend to have throbbing headaches, which get better once the measles skin eruptions appear. (See chapter 4 on colds and coughs for more information on *Euphrasia*).

Bryonia is valuable in treating children with measles when their rash appears late and when the chest is especially affected. *Bryonia* children have a dry, painful cough, chest stitches, soreness of the limbs and body, and sometimes twitching muscles in the face, eyes, and mouth. The muscles ache badly, and the child lies still because it hurts to move, in contrast to the *Gelsemium* child who is just too tired to move. The face is pale and the eyes are red. Constipation and headaches in the front part of the head can accompany the measles. As with all *Bryonia* fevers, dry mouth and an intense thirst

---

Beyond Home Care

Get Medical Care Immediately:

- if your child has a severe headache, excessive lethargy, vomiting, or drowsiness;
- if there is spontaneous bruising or ruptured blood vessels under the skin;
- if there is unexplained bleeding from the rectum, nose, or mouth;
- if there is difficult or rapid breathing.

Get Medical Care Today:

- if an infant less than six months old gets the measles;
- if there is earache;
- if significant coughing lasts more than four days.

See Your Practitioner Soon:

- if the fever and cough do not subside as the rash peaks.

for cold drinks are characteristic. Their symptoms are made worse by motion and warmth and better by cold things and being still.

Pulsatilla is primarily useful in the later stages of measles, when the fever has subsided or has completely gone. The nasal discharge is usually thick and yellowish, and profuse tearing comes from the eyes. The cough is typically dry at night and loose during the day. The *Pulsatilla* child desires cool air, is worse in the heat, and has little thirst. Feelings of queasiness or nausea accompanied by diarrhea may occur. Earaches commonly are experienced too. *Pulsatilla* is also useful when eye problems linger after the measles.

Other less frequently indicated medicines helpful in treating children with measles are:

Ferrum phos.—useful in the initial stages of measles if *Aconite* isn't working, and if *Belladonna* doesn't seem indicated.

Apis—for high fever, much swollen skin, and greatly inflamed eyes and lips worsened by heat. The children are thirstless, tearful, irritable, and delirious.

Kali bi.—useful during the later stages of measles if the earache becomes painful, and swollen glands develop. The children have a sensation of pressure at the root of the nose and perhaps throbbing and burning in the cartilage; they have a rattling cough, and the nose runs with thick, yellow, stringy mucus.

Rhus tox.—for intensely itching rashes and restlessness, which is worse at night and during rest.

Arsenicum—indicated in severe cases of the measles. There is great restlessness, much weakness, delirium, and offensive and exhausting diarrhea.

German Measles

German measles or *rubella* is a harmless disease to children. It is, however, a potential threat to pregnant women since those who contract it during the first three months of pregnancy have a 50–50 chance of delivering an infant who has serious birth defects, including blindness, deafness, heart condition, cleft palate, and mental problems.

German measles is sometimes called the three-day measles. It is shorter and less severe in its symptoms than the "regular" measles which typically lasts seven–ten days. The incubation period ranges from fourteen to twenty-one days. Even though symptoms are apparent for only three days, children with German measles are contagious to others from seven days prior to eruption of the rash and usually for five days after this time.

In a typical case of the German measles, the child becomes mildly ill with a low-grade fever and some nasal discharge about twenty-four to thirty-six hours before the rash develops. There is then painful swelling of the lymph nodes at the back of the head and neck and behind the ears. This swelling may last six or seven days, even beyond the disappearance of the rash. The rash consists of very small, slightly raised spots which begin on the face and spread over the rest of the body within twenty-four hours. Sometimes large areas of the body become flushed and red. The rash reaches the lower legs on the third day as the rash on the face begins to fade.

The above description of symptoms represents the classic form of German measles. Many children, however, have much milder cases. There is often no rash, and their symptoms may be impossible to distinguish from those of colds or other viral infections. Joint pains sometimes occur, though this happens more commonly in adults.

General Home Care

Children with German measles are rarely very sick. They do not need to stay in bed and should be allowed to get up and even go outside on nice days. They should of course stay away from pregnant women.

Homeopathic Medicines

The following homeopathic medicines have been found to be most effective in treating children with German measles: *Aconite, Belladonna, Ferrum phos* and *Pulsatilla*. Read the chapters on measles, fevers, influenzas and the individual materia medica sections for specific information on each medicine's symptomology.

Beyond Home Care

Except for problems resulting from pregnant women getting German measles, there is no evidence that German measles causes significant complications.

Mumps

Mumps is a moderately contagious viral disease with an incubation period lasting fourteen to twenty-one days. The typical symptoms include the characteristic swelling of the parotid salivary glands, which lie just below and in front of the ear lobe, fever ranging from 101° to as high as 105°, loss of appetite, and headache. Other salivary glands under the jaw are sometimes affected. Children are contagious from one day prior to onset of symptoms until the swelling of the salivary glands is completely gone. In adults, mumps may affect other glands such as the ovaries, testes, or pancreas, but sterility rarely occurs.

Nearly half of all children with mumps experience subclinical infections with either no symptoms or only mild symptoms appearing. Measurement of antibodies in the blood can determine if subclinical infections have already established immunity.

Encephalitis, a viral infection of the brain, is an occasional complication of the mumps. Since this condition can be serious, it is especially important to note the symptoms listed in "Beyond Home Care."

General Home Care

Bed rest isn't essential, since mumps is a mild disease. The ill person should keep away from adults who have never had the illness, however. Acid liquids (lemonade, orange juice, ginger ale) and spices should be avoided because they stimulate salivation and increase pain.

Homeopathic Medicines

The indicated dosages for treating people with mumps are the same as those described in the measles section.

Belladonna is the most commonly prescribed medicine for the treatment of mumps. As with so many of *Belladonna's* symptoms, the illness comes on rapidly and violently. The parotid glands are hot and red (they may, in fact, become scarlet red) and are sensitive to touch. There may be burning pain in the throat and shooting pains in the glands, which come and go suddenly. Some spasmodic construction of the throat may occur, especially when the child is drinking or swallowing. There is also a glowing redness of the face. *Belladonna* children are likely to appear dazed or a little delirious. *Belladonna* children occasionally experience sudden lessening of the parotid-gland swelling, which is then followed by a throbbing headache and increased delirium.

Children who need *Phytolacca* have inflammation of the parotid glands and sometimes of the submaxillary glands, which lie under the jaw. The glands may be hard and stony, and the child often experiences a sense of pressure and tension around them. There are often pains that shoot into the ear when the child swallows. The throat feels dry and rough, and there is great difficulty swallowing, especially swallowing anything hot. The face and skin tend to be pale, not *Belladonna's* distinctively red color. *Phytolacca* children's symptoms are worse in cold and wet weather, at night, and with the heat from the bed.

Pulsatilla is considered valuable in treating the later stages of mumps. If the mumps linger and the child is weepy, whiny, thirstless, desires open air, and is worse when warm, *Pulsatilla* should be considered for treatment. *Pulsatilla* is also one of the prime medicines for adults if the mumps become complicated with breast, ovary, or testicle symptoms. *Pulsatilla* children usually have a dry mouth and thickly coated tongue. Most of their symptoms are worse at night and after lying down.

Like those of *Phytolacca,* the symptoms of the *Mercurius* child's mumps may also include swelling of the submaxillary glands as well as the parotids. Some other distinct symptoms *Mercurius* children have are offensive sweat, foul taste on the tongue, foul breath, and much saliva. They usually sweat a lot, especially at night. The affected glands may feel hard to the touch and are tender.

Pilocarpinum is one other important medicine to consider. Drs. Tyler and Burnett, two respected British homeopaths, consider it their best medicine for treating the mumps. There are, however, few differentiating symptoms that indicate its application except profuse sweat, great thirst following the sweat, much salivation, and general weakness. Although there is never just one specific medicine for a disease, Drs. Tyler and Burnett consider *Pilocarpinum* a "near specific."

Other homeopathic medicines to consider in treating children with mumps include:

Aconite—useful during the earliest stages if there's a sudden onset of fever, great restlessness, and a great thirst. The symptoms are worse in warm rooms and better in the open air.

Rhus tox.—appropriate when there is more swelling on the left side; aching in the limbs that is worse at night, during rest, initially during motion but better during continued motion; extreme chilliness and sensitivity to cold; and dry, burning thirst. Frequently, the children have cold sores on the lips.

Bryonia—used with the very irritable, for whom the slightest motion causes pain; even the turning of the head hurts. They also have dry lips and a great thirst for cold water.

Beyond Home Care

Get Medical Care Immediately:

- if there are convulsions, stiffness of the neck, severe headache, or great weakness.

Get Medical Care Today:

- if pain and swelling of the breast, ovaries, or testicles occur;
- if the child has difficulty hearing;
- if the patient has abdominal pains or begins vomiting.

See Your Practitioner Soon

- if you have any uncertainty about your child's illness;
- if your child has recurrent swelling of the parotid gland.

Arsenicum—for severe weakness, chilliness, clammy sweats, anxiousness, and excessive thirst for sips of water. *Arsenicum* is also good if the symptoms have progressed to the breast, ovaries, or testicles. The symptoms are worse after midnight.

Carbo veg.—used when the symptoms have progressed to the breasts, ovaries, or testicles. Other symptoms include chilliness, bluish skin, sluggishness, difficulty getting enough air, lingering fever. Some digestive symptoms, such as gas and bloating, occasionally occur.

Kali bi.—good for fleshy, light-complexioned children or those who have a thick, sticky, stringy nasal discharge accompanying the swollen glands.

Chicken Pox

Chicken pox is an infectious viral disease with an incubation period of ten to twenty-one days. It usually begins with a low-grade fever and a cold. Unlike the flat, barely raised spots typical of measles, chicken pox causes a rash of individual red spots that appear on the child's face, scalp, and torso. At first, these spots look like insect bites, but within hours they develop a small, clear blister in the center. These blisters eventually break and are replaced with a brownish scab. Sometimes the eruptions become infected with bacteria and develop into raw ulcers with pus. Consider your child contagious until all the pox have fully scabbed over.

Children experience chicken pox of different degrees of severity. Some children get only a few spots, and others are literally covered with them. Some may have intense itching; others barely complain. Most children fall somewhere in between these extreme cases. Infrequent complications of chicken pox include encephelitis and pneumonia. Reye's Syndrome (see chapter 3 on fever and influenza) may follow chicken pox.

General Home Care

Bed rest is not required, but you should keep the child away from others since chicken pox is highly contagious. The child should be encouraged not to scratch at the eruptions, for this can cause infection and scarring. Trimming their fingernails is generally a good idea. When bathing children with chicken pox, pat them dry carefully to avoid breaking the blisters or disturbing the scabs. An oatmeal bath sometimes reduces some of the itching. A child's appetite is usually diminished during this illness, and thus it is generally best to prepare small amounts of simple nourishing foods.

Never give aspirin to a child with chicken pox. Although the link has not been definitely proven, aspirin is believed to help trigger Reye's Syndrome, a life-threatening illness, in some children who have had chicken pox.

Homeopathic Medicines

The instructions about the frequency of dosage mentioned in the measles section are applicable here.

A number of homeopaths have stated that *Rhus tox.* is the most effective medicine for treating chicken pox. British homeopath Margaret Tyler referred to it as "the only remedy required," and nineteenth-century American homeopath E. Harris Ruddock said *Rhus tox.* "should be given unless some other remedy is strongly indicated." Despite these declarations, other medicines should also be considered, since the exception to this valuable rule for chicken pox may be your child.

The *Rhus tox.* symptoms include intense itching that grows worse with scratching, at night, and at rest. The eruptions can be large and can have much pus in them. *Rhus tox.* children are very restless and often have great difficulty going to sleep and staying asleep.

Pulsatilla is indicated for children who have its general and mental characteristics. They weep easily but are not very irritable. They have little thirst despite the fever. They are worse in heat and at night and are better in the open air.

The most distinguishing symptom of those who need *Antimonium tart.* is the skin eruption's coming out very slowly and possibly being large. Sometimes the rash is accompanied by a rattling cough and bronchitis.

Other medicines to consider for children with chicken pox include:

Antimonium crudum—for both the physically and the emotionally irritable who cry if washed, touched, or even looked at. Shooting pains occur when pressure is placed on the eruptions.

Arsenicum—for large eruptions with much pus. The eruptions can become open sores. Burning pains accompany extreme chilliness. Pain and itching get worse just prior to and after midnight and in cold.

Belladonna—for chicken pox accompanied by severe headache, flushed face, hot skin, drowsiness, and inability to sleep.

Mercurius—for offensive and profuse sweat and for large eruptions with much pus that sometimes become open sores. The lymph nodes in the neck may get swollen. Symptoms are worse at night and when the patient is hot or cold.

Beyond Home Care

Get Medical Care Immediately:

- if there is severe headache, extreme weakness, convulsions and stiffness of the neck;
- if there is any vomiting, or if respiration is rapid and shallow (Reye's Syndrome must be ruled out);
- if spontaneous bruising or ruptured blood vessels appear under the skin.

Get Medical Care Today:

- if the skin eruption becomes seriously infected;
- if an infant less than one year old gets chicken pox.

See Your Practitioner Soon

- if symptoms linger;
- if the child is breathing much more rapidly than normal.

Note: See also the "Beyond Home Care" section in chapter 4 on colds and coughs for more information.

CHAPTER 6

Earaches

Ear infection is the most common childhood illness other than simple runny nose. Almost every child has had at least one ear infection by the time he or she is six, and for many children and their parents, frequent recurrences of these infections interfere with health and happiness a great deal. Further, the complications of ear infections potentially impair the child's hearing and can retard the acquisition of language skills. Adults sometimes get ear infections too.

There are two main types of ear infections. Infection of the middle ear and eardrum is called *otitis media.* It is the more serious illness and is the type most often meant when a health professional diagnoses an "ear infection." *Otitis externa,* as its name implies, is infection of the outer ear or of the canal that leads to the eardrum. It is actually a skin infection similar to those occurring elsewhere on the body, but it can cause a great deal of ear pain and discharge. We'll discuss each type of ear infection separately.

Not all earaches are due to infections. During a cold many people complain that their ears feel stopped up or that they experience twinges of sharp, brief pains. These symptoms are generally mild. They are due to pressure differences on either side of the eardrum caused by the inflammation and fluid secretion that accompanies a cold. Pressure changes also account for earaches that happen in airplanes or in cars driving up or down a mountain. Some people get earaches whenever they are out in a cold wind or swim in cool water.

Otitis Media

The *middle ear,* the space behind the eardrum, becomes infected during an episode of otitis media. The eustachian tube leads from the middle ear forward and downward, connecting the middle ear to the cavity behind the nose. Normally, the tube opens to allow fluids secreted by mucous cells in the ear to drain into the throat, and to allow pressure in the middle ear to become equalized with the pressure of the atmosphere. At other times, the eustachian tube should be closed to prevent fluids in the nose, which are full of microorganisms, from reaching the middle ear.

Ear infections develop when the eustachian tube opens and closes improperly, allowing germ-laden fluids from the nose and throat to enter but not depart from the middle ear. Inflammation resulting from a cold or allergy may cause this improper function, but in young children sometimes the tube is just too small and short to work properly.

As a middle-ear infection progresses, white blood cells and antibodies are secreted into the tissues and the middle-ear area, where they attack and kill infecting bacteria. As dead bacteria and white cells accumulate, pus forms and puts pressure on the ear drum. The thin eardrum membrane bulges outward, and pain increases as it is stretched. Eventually it may tear, allowing pus to drain to the external auditory canal. This is the way the body expels the pus, and usually a torn eardrum heals rapidly.

The symptoms of acute middle-ear infection are variable. A young child may seem to be in pain, often playing with or pulling at the ears. Older children or adults usually know if something is wrong with the ear, but sometimes even during a severe infection the ear just feels stuffed up. A discharge from the ear may be obvious if the eardrum has ruptured or if the hair around the affected ear is sticky or crusty. Hearing may be less sensitive than usual.

Many children with recurrent ear infections have their own symptom patterns parents learn to recognize in an early stage of the illness. Unusual irritability, emotional sensitivity, or clinginess may accompany ear infection, and sometimes a child's mood changes are the only evidence of the problem. There may be a high fever, but ear infections often occur without any fever at all. Sometimes the child vomits or has diarrhea because of an ear infection, with no sign that something is wrong with the ears. In most cases, if nothing else is responsible, these digestive symptoms clear up rapidly.

The diagnosis of an ear infection depends on accurate visual examination of the eardrum performed with an *otoscope*, a magnifying lens and light that illuminates the drum and external canal through a small speculum that fits into the canal. A normal eardrum has a pearly gray, slightly shiny appearance and looks delicate and translucent. During an infection the most characteristic change is outward bulging of the eardrum due to buildup of pus inside. The eardrum becomes thickened and more opaque and often looks quite red. Redness of the drum, however, may be caused by fever, crying, or cold, and a diagnosis of otitis media should never be made on the basis of a red eardrum alone.

Traditionally, physicians have held that antibiotics effectively treat ear infections and prevent complications. Recently, however, researchers have questioned the value of antibiotic treatment. A carefully performed study of children with otitis media compared the course of the disease in those who received antibiotics and those who were given placebos. The results showed no difference in pain relief, healing time, subsequent hearing impairment, or rate of relapse (Van Buchem 1981). A similar study showed that children given antibiotics early in the course of acute otitis media were significantly (by as much as 2.9 times) more likely to have recurrences than children not treated with antibiotics (Diamant and Diamant 1974). Prior research has shown antibiotics to be more effective than in the above studies, but it seems clear that they are not the cure-all they were thought to be.

Be watchful if otitis media is diagnosed. Serious acute complications of middle-ear infection are rare but do occur. These include *mastoiditis*, infection of the bony area just behind the ear. Be alert for any redness, tenderness, pain, or swelling in this area and report these symptoms immediately to your practitioner. Mastoiditis can become a chronic problem and result in hearing loss and erosion of the bone.

Meningitis and other infections of the central nervous system may result from acute otitis media if the infection spreads through the blood stream to bony structures. Symptoms of these problems include severe or persistent headache, stiff neck, persistent vomiting, and marked change in mood or alertness.

The most common complications of middle-ear infections are the chronic ear problems that often follow. *Serous otitis media,* accumulation of a translucent noninfectious fluid in the middle ear, interferes with normal motion of the eardrum and the tiny middle-ear bones so that hearing is reduced. Homeopathic constitutional treatment is often effective with chronic serous otitis. Antihistamines and decongestants are worthless, though they are often prescribed. Conventional treatment for persistent hearing loss due to serous otitis involves surgical insertion of polyethylene tubes into the eardrum to allow drainage of middle-ear fluid. These tubes seem to improve treated ears' hearing for a few months, and this may be very important to the child who is at a crucial stage of language development. Research has shown, however, that there is no long-term improvement in hearing when tubes are inserted, and eardrums in which tubes have been placed tend to become scarred. We believe that the tubes should be inserted for serous otitis only when there is a significant, documented hearing problem, when the risks of the surgery are clearly understood, and when the goal of treatment is improved hearing within a short period.

General Home Care

General recommendations for any infectious illness apply to people with acute middle-ear infections; they should rest, have plenty of liquids, and be comforted. A heating pad or hot washcloth applied to the ear may help reduce pain.

To help prevent ear infection, avoid nursing or bottle feeding children when they are in a lying position; gravity may allow milk or juice to run into the eustachian tubes, encouraging infection. Allergies may predispose an individual to ear infection by causing inflammation and fluid buildup; identification of the substances that trigger allergic reactions for that person can be helpful.

Beyond Home Care

See "Beyond Home Care" that follows "Otitis Externa."

Otitis Externa

External ear infections are essentially skin infections involving the canal that leads from the outer ear to the eardrum. The symptoms of external ear infections often include much ear pain and throbbing due to inflammation. The pain is characteristically aggravated by moving the outer ear, so a helpful way to differentiate between middle ear and external ear infections is to pull on the earlobe. Both types of ear infections can be present at the same time, so you should still use the guidelines in "Beyond Home Care" to decide if medical consultation is needed. Often the ear canal is quite itchy during an external ear infection. If you look into the canal, you can see that it is red and scaly or wet, and a thick discharge may be present. There is usually no fever or general symptoms of illness.

External ear infections do not endanger the organs of hearing, although the discharge and swelling may reduce hearing for a time. As with all skin infections, there is some small danger that the infection will spread aggressively. Rapidly spreading redness or swelling of the outer ear or nearby skin is a danger sign, as is onset of fever.

General Home Care

Gently wash out the accumulated scaling and discharge by placing a piece of cotton soaked in dilute vinegar (half water/half vinegar) or Burow's solution (available at drug stores) in the ear canal and leaving it for eight to twelve hours. Make sure you can pull the cotton out easily again. Then briefly rinse the canal with warm water, using a bulb syringe. Let the ear drain after this, but put in a drop or two of the vinegar solution every eight hours or so.

Homeopathic Medicines

The following descriptions apply to children with ear infections, but the indications for adults are the same. Most of the descriptions of physical-exam findings (color and shape of the eardrum) apply to otitis media, but all the other symptoms are applicable to those with both middle-ear infections and otitis externa. You can also use these descriptions to treat the person with a earache due to something other than infection.

Many of these medicines share similar symptoms. For example, *Silica, Hepar sulph.,* and *Mercurius* are all equally indicated by the presence of painfully swollen lymph nodes in the head and neck that commonly occur with ear infections. If no medicine is strongly indicated, start with either *Pulsatilla,* if the child is more clingy than usual, or *Mercury,* if the child is somewhat irritable or severe pain is the predominant feature of the illness.

Give a dose of the medicine you choose every three to six hours, depending on the severity of the symptoms, but stop as soon as you notice definite improvement. Repeat the medicine only when symptoms begin to get worse again, or if no further improvement has occured after twelve hours. Switch to another medicine if you see no improvement within twelve to twenty-four hours after beginning treatment.

Belladonna is the most commonly indicated homeopathic medicine during the early stages of an ear infection or earache, especially when the illness begins suddenly with few prior cold symptoms. Within an hour or two the child is in intense pain. He may have had a watery runny nose for a short while, but the mucus isn't cloudy, colored, or thick. The outer ear, ear canal, or eardrum may be bright red, but pus hasn't formed and the eardrum is still normally shaped. A sudden high fever (with the characteristics described in chapter 3) often begins about the same time as the earache. The ear pain may extend down into the neck, and there may be associated sore-throat or facial pain.

Ferrum phos. is used in much the same way in the early stages of suddenly occuring earaches not yet accompanied by pus formation. The onset is not quite as sudden, the fever is not so high, and the overall condition of the child is a little less intense.

Chamomilla is indicated chiefly by the effects of the illness on the child's mood, and less so by particular symptoms. Children for whom *Chamomilla* is indicated are extremely irritable. They scream and cry angrily, do not want to be touched, and can't be comforted. They may ask for things that they then reject, and they are likely to hit you for crossing them at all or for no apparent reason. Sometimes the child can be calmed by being carried. The earache generally doesn't come on as quickly as in the *Belladonna* case, but the pain is severe and the child may scream. The child may be made worse when stooping or bending over and improved by warmth or being wrapped in warm covers. A discharge from the ear is less typical of *Chamomilla* than of other medicines discussed later. There is usually a watery runny nose and, less often, a very thick discharge. As with *Belladonna*, the nasal mucus is usually not colored. Whatever the particular symptoms, though, be sure to consider *Chamomilla* for the child who is in severe pain, especially if he is extremely irritable.

Another commonly effective medicine is *Pulsatilla*. In contrast to *Chamomilla*, it is indicated for children who are sweet, placid, loving, and mild during the earache. The *Pulsatilla* child may be irritable, but the irritability is weak and whiny, not violent as is the *Chamomilla* or *Hepar* anger. *Pulsatilla* children want to be held and cuddled and are comforted when given affection. They too may scream with the pain but are just as likely to weep piteously. *Pulsatilla* is more frequently indicated for ear infections that develop after cold symptoms have been persistent for a few days. The nasal discharge has become thick and yellow-to-green in color. Though pain may be fairly severe, sometimes there seems to be no pain at all. Examination often shows a red, swollen eardrum and a buildup of pus in the middle ear. A thick yellow-green discharge may be seen at the external canal. The pain is typically worse at night and in a warm room. There may be a sensation of pressure in the ear. The child may or may not be feverish but tends to feel uncomfortably warm and wants fresh air. She is noticeably less thirsty than usual, even with a high fever. In any case, the strongest indication for *Pulsatilla* is the characteristic mildness and clinginess of the child.

Lycopodium is commonly indicated during any stage of earaches. Children who need this medicine are irritable and fussy, though their tempers are less extreme than with *Chamomilla*. They are dissatisfied, "bratty," and bossy, but are likely also to be insecure and may fear the dark or being alone. Thirst is likely to be diminished. The earache is most often worse on the right side.

Silica is also indicated for the middle and later stages of a cold accompanied by an ear infection. The child who needs *Silica* also is mild and whimpering but is less loving and less interested in affection than the *Pulsatilla* child. Also characteristic of children for whom *Silica* is indicated are marked physical weakness and tiredness. The illness seems to have really worn them out. They are definitely chilly and want warm covering. They may have sweat about the head or on the hands or feet. If there is pain in the ear, it may be intense but usually not as severe as the pain of some of the other medicines. It tends to occur at night and is made worse by cold applications, moving, sitting for a long time, and noise. *Silica* is the remedy most prominently indicated for pain behind the ear in the region of the mastoid, though many other medicines also cover this complaint. There may be itching in the ear (also symptoms of *Hepar sulph.* and *Mercurius*) or a stopped-up sensa-

---

Beyond Home Care

Get Medical Care Immediately:

- if earache is accompanied by severe weakness, loss of alertness, severe headache, or stiffness of the neck.

Get Medical Care Today:

- if a baby begins to pull or rub her ears;
- for any definite earache or any ear discharge in a child under seven years old;
- for anyone with severe earache, especially if it's accompanied by fever or ear discharge;
- if there is tenderness or redness in the bony area behind the ear;
- if there is sudden, significant decrease in hearing—with or without pain.

See Your Practitioner Soon:

- if an older child or adult has had mild ear pain or discharge lasting longer than one or two weeks;
- if mild hearing loss lasts longer than two weeks.

tion. The examination may show inflammation and pus formation, and there may be drainage of pus or watery fluid from the ear. A nasal discharge, of any character, often accompanies the infection. The physical symptoms indicating *Hepar sulph.* are similar to those of *Silica* but more intense. Again, this is a remedy best given during the middle and late stages of colds and ear infections, when a thick, colored nasal discharge often precedes or accompanies the earache and when inflammation in the middle ear has progressed to the point that pus has formed. You should think of *Hepar* when the child is intensely, even violently irritable about everything. Although this emotional state is similar to that described for *Chamomilla,* the child is a little less expressive, is less prone to scream constantly or hit, doesn't have such a strong aversion to being held, and is less likely to throw away things she asked for. But the *Hepar* child lets you know, in no uncertain terms, that she is angry. *Hepar* is indicated for children who are very chilly—cold air or coldness of any sort makes them uncomfortable and provokes symptoms. The child wants the heat turned up, and she wants lots of blankets. The earache is usually severe and is worse at night. It is also made worse by cold air, open air, and cold applications and is improved by warmth and bundling up.

Mercurius is also indicated for earaches after pus formation has occurred. The child needing *Mercurius* is somewhat irritable and may act impulsively or hastily, or he may be less alert than when normal. He may be generally bothered by heat or cold or both, but this particular earache is typically made worse by warmth, especially the warmth of the bed. Pain is worse at night. Characteristic *Mercurius* symptoms also include profuse and offensive perspiration, head sweats, increased salivation, bad breath, puffiness of the tongue, and trembling or twitching.

CHAPTER 7

Sore Throats

A SORE THROAT may be the sign of a viral or bacterial infection, but just as commonly it results from a postnasal drip or simply from dryness of the throat. Most sore throats, even when they result from infections, are self-limited symptoms that the body can heal on its own. Medical practitioners use throat cultures to determine whether *Streptococcus* bacteria are involved; usually, no attempt to identify other specific germs is made.

Noninfectious Sore Throats

Mucus trickling down the back of the nose and into the throat often causes enough irritation to produce pain. Postnasal drip can be a problem for those with acute colds or acute attacks of allergies like hay fever or reactions to cat fur. It can also trouble those who have chronic nasal congestion due to allergy. People with acute symptoms can be treated at home according to the guidelines in chapters 4 and 12 on colds and allergies, but those with chronic or recurrent symptoms should be treated by a professional homeopath.

Sore throats are also commonly the result of dryness caused by open-mouth breathing or artificially heated air.

Viral and Non-Strep Bacterial Infections of the Throat

A substantial number of infectious sore throats are precipitated by the same viruses that cause the common cold. Recent research, however, has shown that bacteria other than *Streptococcus* are much more frequently involved in sore throats than had been thought. Symptoms accompanying both viral and bacterial throat infections are various. Pain may be minimal or intense; fever, swollen lymph nodes, and pus in the throat may or may not be present. Cold symptoms often occur.

Less commonly, other viruses infect the throat with more severe symptoms. Both herpangina and true herpes viral throat infections may cause marked general symptoms and small blisters or sores on the throat tissues. Mononucleosis, another viral infection, may cause severe sore throats. We discuss mononucleosis in more detail later in this chapter.

Sore throats that result from infections caused by viruses or nonstrep bacteria are not very serious. They clear up on their own, though the patient with mononucleosis may be sick for quite a while. Other kinds of bacteria that infect the throat produce self-limited illnesses and rarely lead to serious complications.

Conventional medicine offers no treatment for viral infections associated with sore throat. Antibiotics are useless and can be risky. At this time there are no simple tests to detect nonstrep bacterial sore throats. Since they don't cause any serious problems and since they clear up by themselves, antibiotic treatment is unnecessary.

Strep Throat

"Strep" refers to a particular type of bacteria, the group A beta-hemolytic *Streptococcus*. Although a person with a strep throat is often sicker and has a higher fever and more pain than one with a viral sore throat, the disease itself is not serious; the symptoms clear up within a few days. Cold symptoms and coughs are less likely to accompany a strep throat than a viral sore throat. Scarlet fever may occur, but this is simply strep throat accompanied by a rash, and the treatment of a person with scarlet fever is no different from that of simple strep throat. The main reason for the concern about strep throats is that they can, though rarely do, lead to serious illnesses, including kidney inflammation and rheumatic fever.

The person with a kidney disease resulting from a prior strep infection becomes quite ill, but usually recovers without any permanent ill effects. On the other hand, rheumatic fever can lead to permanent heart damage to one or more of the valves of the heart. Rheumatic fever has become quite rare, but its prevention is still taken seriously.

Rheumatic fever can be prevented if all the strep germs are killed within the first ten to twelve days of the infection. Often, the body's own defenses have eradicated the strep within that time. Still, to be safe and to prevent spread of the infection to others, when children's throat cultures show positive signs of strep throat, pediatric authorities recommend they receive penicillin or other appropriate antibiotic treatment. In order to prevent rheumatic fever, antibiotic treatment must be begun within the first nine days of the symptoms.

According to many studies, antibiotics do not relieve discomfort or shorten the course of the symptoms unless the treatment is begun during the first twenty-four hours. This period has usually passed by the time a strep infection is diagnosed. Also, various studies have shown that even the proper use of orally administered penicillin fails to eradicate strep bacteria in up to 30% of those treated.

Although they are not a panacea, antibiotics do successfully eliminate the strep bacteria in the majority of cases. We recommend children receive penicillin or other appropriate antibiotics along with the homeopathic treatment if a throat culture shows strep infection, since most cases of rheumatic fever occur in children five to fifteen years old. Any child with a family history of rheumatic fever should definitely receive antibiotics. Adults in generally good health with no family history of rheumatic fever need not take penicillin unless they will be exposing others to the disease. People of any age who themselves have had rheumatic fever must take antibiotics preventively from the onset of any significant sore throat, even before culture results are known.

Homeopathic treatment of those with strep is often very effective in helping the person heal from the illness. You may use homeopathic medicine even while taking antibiotics, and you can certainly begin homeopathic treatment while you're waiting for the results of the throat culture.

Mononucleosis

"Mono" is a viral infection of the whole system and is most common in ten-to-thirty-five year olds. Symptoms often include a very painful sore throat and red, swollen tonsils, sometimes spotted with white material. The lymph nodes, especially those towards the back of the neck, are always swollen. Mono is like the flu. The person feels exhausted and achy and has a fever. But mono lasts longer than the flu, and the sore throat is worse. Mono may also be accompanied by cough, hepatitis (liver inflammation), swelling of the spleen, or symptoms affecting the nervous system. A blood test is required to confirm the existence of mono. There is no orthodox medical treatment for mono, and it usually resolves on its own in two to four weeks, though it may last up to three months.

Epiglottitis

The *epiglottis* is the flap of tissue that covers the entrance to the larynx; when one swallows, it prevents food from getting into the tube leading to the lungs. Rarely, the epiglottis becomes infected by baceria, resulting in a serious medical emergency, since swelling of the epiglottis may totally block the windpipe. The symptoms—severe sore throat, sense of constriction, and marked fever—begin suddenly. As the swelling worsens, swallowing becomes so difficult that drooling is extremely noticeable. Struggling to pull air into the lungs past the obstruction, the patient often sits leaning forward and open-mouthed. Epiglottitis requires immediate emergency treatment from a hospital.

General Home Treatment

Sore throats caused or aggravated by dryness are often relieved simply by reducing room heat, running a humidifier, and remembering to take frequent sips of liquid. Gargling with warm salt water, lemon juice and honey in warm water, or dilute apple cider vinegar temporarily relieves sore throat pain. Throat lozenges may help too. Sucking on a 100 mg or 500 mg tablet of vitamin C may be soothing, but be careful not to irritate the tongue or throat. If you are being treated with homeopathic medicine, however, do not take lozenges containing menthol or eucalyptus, since these substances may interfere with the action of the medicine.

Home treatment for mononucleosis is the same as for other sore throats or for flus. Vigorous activity must be avoided, since the spleen is vulnerable to rupture.

Homeopathic Medicines

The person with a sore throat should receive a dose of your selected medicine every six to eight hours for about two days. Stop as soon as improvement is definite. Since all medicines listed here cover swollen lymph nodes and scarlet fever rash, these two symptoms are not repeated in each remedy description.

When a person has a sore throat, *Belladonna* is the first medicine to think of. During the first twenty-four hours, if the pain has come on suddenly, particularly if it is accompanied by fever and flushed skin, *Belladonna* is the likely medicine. The throat is very red and may be quite swollen, but little or no pus is evident. The tongue may have a "strawberry" appearance as in scarlet fever. Swallowing, especially swallowing liquids, makes the throat pain worse, and the patient may have an aversion to drinking. There may also be a great sense of dryness in the throat.

Aconite should be considered after sudden onset of not only sore throat and high fever but also thirst (the *Belladonna* patient is not so thirsty and may be actually averse to liquids). The condition may have begun after exposure to cold or drafts. *Aconite*'s other characteristic mental symptoms may be present.

Arsenicum should be considered when the general symptoms of the medicine are evident: chilliness even during fever, thirst, and restlessness combined with fatigue. Most typically, the throat pain is burning in character. Warm drinks relieve the pain, whereas swallowing, cold drinks, or exposure to the cold make it worse.

The *Rhus tox.* person has a painfully sore throat that is made better by warm drinks and warmth in general. The pain in the throat is usually worse in the morning. The pain often begins after straining the throat while speaking or singing or after exposure to cold, wet weather. Sometimes the pain is worst upon first swallowing and then decreases with later swallowing. The *Rhus tox.* patient is very restless but is less tired and more achy than the *Arsenicum* patient. He may be anxious, irritable, and weepy.

Lycopodium sore throats are typically worse on the right side or begin on the right side and spread to the left. The pain may be relieved by either warm or cold drinks, whereas being in cold air may make it worse. There may be pain extending up into the ears. In general, the illness doesn't begin particularly suddenly, and usually the patient isn't terribly sick. She typically wants fresh air. The symptoms in general, sometimes including the sore throat, may be worse in the late afternoon, between 4 and 8 P.M. in classic cases.

When the sore throat is severe and is accompanied by fever and weakness, *Mercurius* may be indicated. The throat is red and swollen, and pus or other white or yellow material may be seen on the tonsils or walls of the throat. The *Mercurius* patient can be generally sensitive to both heat and cold. Becoming cold aggravates the throat pain, but a warm bed may also make it worse. Liquids of any temperature aren't known to influence the symptoms particularly. The sore throat tends to be more painful at night. A classic *Mercurius* sore-throat symptom is the tendency to salivate and drool. The pillow may be wet or more frequent swallowing may be noticeable. The tongue often looks or feels swollen or puffy, and at times the teeth make imprints on the tongue. The breath may smell bad. There may be cold symptoms such as thick, greenish or yellow mucus draining from the nose.

Hepar sulph. is similar to *Mercurius* in severity of infection. Pus has formed and the throat and tonsils are very swollen. Often the person says he feels something stuck in his throat like a splinter (*Lachesis* and *Apis* may also have this symptom, though less characteristically). The patient is irritable and easily angered. Chilliness is a predominant symptom, and both the general condition and the sore throat are definitely aggravated by exposure to cold. Warm drinks and warmth in general soothe the sore throat. The pain may extend to the ears.

Lachesis is particularly useful to those with painfully swollen throats that are worse on the left side or begin there and spread to the right. Drinking, especially drinking warm liquids, makes the pain worse (sometimes cold drinks bring some relief), but solid foods are more difficult to swallow than liquids. Usually the symptoms are made worse by warmth in general, and the pain is often worse in the morning, especially upon waking, and during the day. The throat is sensitive to touch, and clothing around the neck may cause pain or a choking sensation. A *sensation* of swelling in the throat is a strong symptom of *Lachesis* (as well as *Hepar, Rhus tox.,* and *Sulphur*).

When the pain of a sore throat is stinging in character, *Apis* may be the medicine, particularly if the pain is made better by cold drinks and worse by warm ones. The throat, tonsils, and tongue are swollen and characteristically appear as though they were filled with water. The burning or stinging pain is worse in heat and with warm drinks, better in coolness or with cold drinks. There is generally an absence of thirst.

Phytolacca should be given when there is much aching in the body along with the fever and when the sore throat is worse with warm drinks. The appearance of the throat may be dark red or even purplish or bluish, and the glands are swollen. The pain may shoot up to the ears, particularly during swallowing. People who need *Phytolacca* tend to have an incessant desire to swallow, despite the fact that it is painful to do so. They are cold and like to be covered, but they still may feel chilly. Their body aches may cause them to be restless, but these pains are worse during motion. One rare but distinctive feature of people who need *Phytolacca* is an acute pain felt at the base of the tongue when protruded.

Sulphur should be considered when a sore throat lingers or when the indicated medicine is not working, as long as some of the *Sulphur* general and particular symptoms match the person's own. There is much burning pain in the throat, with dryness of the mucous membranes, diminished appetite, and increased thirst. Despite the burning, the pain is better when the patient drinks warm liquids. The pain in the throat can also be stitching, pressing, or cutting. A sensation like a lump, splinter, or hair in the throat may be experienced. The general symptoms of *Sulphur*—particularly discomfort from warmth, general lethargy, and offensive breath, sweat, and discharges—are important in determining when to use it.

Beyond Home Care

Get Medical Care Immediately:

- if there is a severe sore throat and great difficulty swallowing, or if there is much drooling or difficulty breathing.

Get Medical Care Today:

- if there is swelling of the region around the tonsils to the extent that it is bulging or pushing the uvula to one side.
- if a sore throat is accompanied by a fever and a red rash that feels like sandpaper.
- if a child has a significant sore throat, or a sore throat and fever, for more than a day or two. Adults can safely wait a few days longer.
- if there is white or yellowish material on the tonsils or throat.
- if a person who previously had rheumatic fever gets a sore throat.

CHAPTER **8**

Digestive Problems

FOR MANY people, the gastrointestinal tract is the first system of the body to develop symptoms when stress levels rise. Many nonserious digestive conditions can be cared for at home with homeopathic medicine or other home treatment measures. These include the common causes of vomiting, diarrhea, and abdominal pain. Appropriate homeopathic medicines for all of these conditions are listed together. Vomiting and diarrhea are the most common causes of dehydration, although it can occur during any acute illness. Therefore, we include a section on the prevention and recognition of dehydration in this chapter. We have a few comments about the frequently troublesome indigestion and constipation complaints, for which we think simple home-care measures usually suffice. We also cover the homeopathic treatment of motion sickness.

Along with playing many other physiological roles, the liver is an important digestive organ. *Hepatitis*, acute liver disease, always requires professional medical attention, but you may still want to use home treatment with homeopathic medicines to speed the healing process.

Gastroenteritis and Other Causes of Vomiting and Diarrhea

Often called "stomach flu," *acute gastroenteritis* is the generic medical term for the common infectious illness of the gastrointestinal tract. The symptoms include some combination of vomiting, diarrhea, and abdominal cramping. Acute gastroenteritis is usually virus related, but you can also contract bacterial gastroenteritis by eating spoiled food (food poisoning). Both types of gastroenteritis are short-term, self-limited illnesses that get better once the body neutralizes the infecting germs or bacterial toxins. They can, however, make you feel very sick, often with fever and general achiness in addition to the digestive symptoms.

The main risk with these illnesses is that prolonged vomiting or diarrhea may exhaust reserves of body fluid before healing takes place. Children and especially babies are at much greater risk of serious fluid loss than adults. Today worldwide, more infant deaths result from dehydration caused by diarrhea than from any other condition.

The chief digestive symptoms of gastroenteritis, vomiting and diarrhea, can also be caused by other conditions. Some of these can be treated at home, but others require medical assistance.

Vomiting

Although it is decidedly an uncomfortable experience, vomiting is an important and effective defense mechanism. It allows the body to rid itself of poisons and germs, and it can remove food the gastrointestinal tract is not working well enough to properly digest and absorb. Nausea usually precedes vomiting and serves as a useful warning that all is not well with the digestive system and that eating would not be a good idea.

The most common cause of vomiting in any age group is gastroenteritis. Vomiting, especially children's, may also be caused by infection elsewhere in the body. Conditions like ear infections, colds and flus, urinary infections, and more serious illnesses can all lead to vomiting, sometimes before the symptoms of the "real" illness are apparent. Usually vomiting associated with other infections is mild and only happens once or twice, but if the vomiting itself requires treatment, the advice in the "General Home Care" section should be followed. Homeopathic treatment should be based on the overall symptom picture no matter what the name of the disease. If a cold or ear infection is accompanied by significant vomiting, try to find the one remedy that best covers all of the person's symptoms.

Children vomit easily. Their digestive tracts are generally more sensitive than adults'. Psychological upset as well as eating too much food or too many sweets may make a child vomit once or twice, whereas an adult might just feel queasy.

Many babies spit up frequently after nursing or bottle feeding. The milk comes up because the muscular valve that should close off the bottom of the esophagus is not yet fully developed. Babies can spit up what seems to be quite a lot of their food and still grow and gain weight adequately. As long as the vomited material is simply "burped up" and doesn't come up forcefully, and as long as the child seems comfortable and is gaining enough weight, there is no cause for concern; the condition eventually corrects itself.

Other uncommon conditions associated with vomiting in both children and adults may be serious or even life-threatening. We will indicate these in "Beyond Home Care."

Diarrhea

Diarrhea is defined as an increase in both the frequency and looseness of stools. "Frequency" is important because even a very loose bowel movement is of little immediate significance if it only occurs once or twice a day. Diarrhea, like vomiting, is another way the body can rapidly eliminate germs, toxins, and irritants from the gastrointestinal tract. When the intestinal linings are infected or when poisons or irritants are present, absorption of fluids and nutrients is reduced, and the muscular walls of the intestine contract more vigorously and more rapidly. The result that you are aware of is a loose or liquid stool, but the body has accomplished the disposal of harmful materials.

Acute diarrhea, like vomiting, most often occurs with gastroenteritis or along with other infectious illnesses such as ear infection or flu; again, this is more common in children. The main concern with diarrhea caused by these conditions is excessive loss of body fluids, especially in children (see the section on dehydration below for more information about this problem). Otherwise, home treatment and careful observation are usually all that are necessary.

Breast-fed babies usually have very loose stools as frequently as eight times a day or so. Once the child is started on formulas or solids, the stools generally get firmer and come less often. Children have more sensitive digestive tracts than adults and may have diarrhea after fairly minor psychological or dietary upsets. No treatment other than avoidance of irritating foods and relief of stress is necessary in these cases.

Diarrhea from being infected with one-celled, microscopic animals (*Giardia lamblia* and *Entomeba histolytica* cause the majority of these cases) is becoming increasingly common in the United States. Sexual contact with an infected person, drinking contaminated water (*Giardia* can be found in many streams and lakes), and poor hygiene among infected children or during their diaper changes spread these infections. Travellers to foreign countries are especially vulnerable to these infections. Symptoms vary from none at all to severe and debilitating diarrhea. When a family member has a suspected or confirmed infection, it must be followed by a medical professional, but you may use homeopathic medicines in addition to other prescribed treatments to help restore health to the intestinal tract.

Other causes of acute and chronic diarrhea may be serious and should not be treated at home. Again, check our "Beyond Home Care" section.

General Home Care

When acute vomiting or diarrhea occur, the best way to help the body heal is to carefully limit what you eat and drink. Food and even liquids irritate the inflamed linings of the stomach and intestines, attracting more fluid from the blood stream and touching off renewed bouts. Adults and children should begin home care by spending six to twelve hours without food or drink of any kind.

When the symptoms have calmed down a bit, try taking clear liquids in sips or teaspoonfuls to replace the water and minerals the body is losing and to provide some simple sugars for energy. Fruit juice or flat soft drinks diluted to half water, vegetable broth (simmer mixed vegetables in water for ten or fifteen minutes, then strain) or rice water (use an excess of water to cook rice) are all good choices. Broths or soup stocks made with oil or animal fat should be avoided, as should milk. Gradually increase the amount of clear liquids over a day or two, and then begin trying low-fiber foods such as white rice or toast, low-fat yogurt or cottage cheese, or bananas.

Younger children and babies do not have the fluid reserves of adults, so begin replacing their fluid losses at once. The breast-fed baby should continue its nursing, but all other liquids and solids should be discontinued. If a baby has been vomiting, you should try to reduce the breast milk taken per feeding to avoid touching off more vomiting. If diarrhea is present without vomiting, offer the breast frequently and allow the baby to drink as much as she wants.

Babies on formula and young children who have been weaned should receive clear liquids only (as outlined above) from the time the symptoms become apparent. Discontinue formula and milk products. If the child has been vomiting, it is vital that you get her to hold down some fluids to replace those lost. You may have to start with tiny amounts of liquids, perhaps only a tablespoon every fifteen minutes. Children who have diarrhea can drink fluids only when they feel they want them. Be sure to offer them frequently, even when the child doesn't ask. If the child refuses to drink, you'll have to watch carefully for signs of dehydration.

Begin reintroducing the child's normal diet as the symptoms improve, usually a day or two after they began.

Dehydration

The body is composed of mostly water; the brain, the kidneys, various hormones, and other systems all work together in intricate harmony to maintain the body's vital-fluid balance. Water is constantly lost in the urine, in perspiration, in the stool, and in water vapor that leaves the lungs when we breathe. In healthy people with an average activity level, about half the body's water loss occurs through the skin and lungs. Illness increases these losses since perspiration and deep, rapid breathing accompany fevers, repiratory illnesses, vomiting and diarrhea, and any type of stress.

Although there are powerful regulatory mechanisms that conserve fluids and minerals if intake is low or losses are high, and although there are sizeable reserves of fluid in the body, the body is not always able to cope with low intake or excessive loss of fluids. Once fluid levels drop below the necessary minimum, function of many crucial systems of the body becomes impaired. This is *dehydration.* Mineral losses that occur when large amounts of fluids are lost through vomiting, diarrhea, and such may also cause serious problems, since minerals play necessary roles in such vital physiological functions as contraction of muscles, transmission of nerve impulses, and regulation of heartbeat.

Babies under six months old are at the greatest risk of dehydrating and suffering dehydration's severe consequences. Their metabolic rate is high, their kidneys don't retain water so well yet, and they lose greater proportions of water per unit of weight than adults do.

The risk of dehydration decreases with age, but it can happen to anyone if fluid losses are great enough. Older people, who may have impaired kidney function and reduced fluid reserves, are also at increased risk.

General Home Care

Anyone with an acute illness should drink some extra liquid. If there is little fever and no respiratory symptoms, the increase need not be large—a couple of extra glasses of water or juice a day is fine. If fever, congestion of the nose, or cough are present, another couple of glasses should be taken. Instructions for making sure the person with vomiting or diarrhea gets enough fluid are given in this section under gastroenteritis. Anyone who is sick, but particularly

---

Beyond Home Care

Get Medical Care Immediately:

- if the mouth or eyes are truly dry (no saliva or tears)
- if there is loss of normal skin texture: if skin is pinched up and does not immediately snap back into place
- if the eyes appear sunken
- in babies, if the soft spot at the top of the head is sunken
- if the quantitiy of urine is definitely and markedly reduced

children and elderly people, should be offered liquids every hour or two, since they may be just too tired or woozy to respond to thirst.

Anyone with severe vomiting or diarrhea, and babies with any degree of these symptoms or decreased thirst with their illness, should be closely watched for signs of dehydration. The first indication that fluid losses are too great is dryness of the mouth and eyes—as long as the person still has tears and saliva, he is not yet dehydrated. As dehydration worsens, later signs are (1) loss of the normal texture of the skin (if you pinch up some skin it does not immediately snap back into place); (2) sunken eyes; and (3) in babies, a sunken "soft spot" at the top of the head. A definite reduction in the quantity of urine is also a bad sign. Immediate medical attention should be obtained as soon as you notice dry mouth or lack of tears.

Abdominal Pain and Indigestion

Abdominal pain is often one of the symptoms of acute gastroenteritis, but more often the immediate cause of acute cramping pains in the abdomen is indigestion and gas. Indigestion is a vague term but we use it to mean all the minor gastrointestinal symptoms: heartburn, queasiness, burping, gas, and so on.

Acute bouts of such symptoms are usually the result of bad diet or psychological stress. Eating too much in general, eating too many foods at one meal, or eating too rapidly may cause just as much trouble as particular problem foods or beverages. The nerves that regulate the contractions of the intestinal muscles are part of the same system that controls the body's "fight or flight" response to stress, so stress can also upset the digestive tract and cause indigestion. The symptoms of indigestion are usually only uncomfortable nuisances, but at times gas and cramping can cause intense pain.

There are a number of more serious causes for acute abdominal pain, and even experienced surgeons can have trouble diagnosing the problem. But if the pain is not extreme, and as long as there are not worrisome accompanying symptoms, you can treat the person at home for a few hours. If you suspect appendicitis, read on.

Appendicitis

The appendix is a "blind alley" outpouching about half an inch long that hangs from the place where the small and large intestines join. Long thought to have no function in the body, the appendix is now known to contain lymphatic tissue and to play a role in the immune system of the gastrointestinal tract. It may be a kind of filter that helps protect the large intestine from harmful microbes.

This makes questionable the common practice of removing the appendix "preventively" during abdominal surgery for other reasons. One study demonstrated a slight increase in cancer of the large intestine in those whose healthy appendixes had been removed surgically as compared with those who still had theirs.

Of course, the appendix can become diseased. When it gets clogged with fecal material, it may become inflamed and swollen, and a bacterial infection may develop in its walls. As the swelling stretches the walls, pain becomes severe. Eventually the appendix bursts, and inflammation and infection spreads throughout the abdomen. This complication, called *peritonitis*, is extremely dangerous. Appendicitis must therefore be diagnosed before the appendix bursts.

As with other causes of abdominal pain, appendicitis is hard to diagnose. The most typical pattern of symptoms runs as follows: After a short period of disinterest in food, and perhaps a mild episode of vomiting, the person with appendicitis begins to feel pain in the area of the navel. Within another few hours the pain moves from the center of the abdomen and becomes localized in the right lower section of the abdomen. Touching the painful area increases the pain and, as inflammation progresses, the muscles of the abdomen become tense and hard. There may be a fever of a degree or two over normal, and the person may be constipated.

There are other conditions that mimic this pattern of symptoms, but you should still be extremely wary of appendicitis if you see this pattern. When the classic symptom pattern is apparent, it is not such a problem as when appendicitis causes different symptoms, however. Some authorities estimate that the "typical" pattern occurs in only one-fifth of the cases. Young children and older people are especially likely to have confusing symptoms. The diagnosis of appendicitis can be made more definite by careful examination of the abdomen and rectum and with blood tests, but the diagnosis is never confirmed until during surgery.

General Home Care

The milder symptoms of indigestion are best treated at home by letting them pass and refraining from doing anything that might aggravate the system further. You may do well to put off eating altogether, but certainly avoid spices, coffee, alcohol, and fatty or oily foods. Herb teas such as peppermint or raspberry leaf are a good means of helping relieve gas. Changing position frequently or walking slowly may help gas move more freely.

Relaxation exercises and other ways of effectively dealing with stress are briefly discussed in chapter 11 on headaches. They are a good idea if your symptoms were brought on by stress, and even when this isn't the case, they sometimes help relieve indigestion or abdominal pain.

If you have definite abdominal pain, avoid solid foods and take only clear liquids. As long as you don't have diarrhea or vomiting, plain water is best. Some people get relief using a hot water bottle or heating pad, applying slight pressure, or bending double.

For cases of mild to moderate abdominal pain, we think that it makes sense to watch and wait for a few hours before seeking medical care. Most often the pain will pass, and in those few cases of serious problems the wait won't hurt. Don't hesitate to try an appropriate homeopathic medicine while waiting for the seriousness of the problem to become clear. Even if you eventually need more extreme medical measures, the correct medicine may well help your body heal more rapidly.

Homeopathic Medicines

Most of the medicines listed here may be useful for people with any combination of digestive symptoms, including vomiting, diarrhea, or pain. Give a dose of the best-indicated medicine every hour (during intense pain or incessant retching) to every twelve hours (if vomiting or diarrhea is mild). Severe symptoms should improve rapidly, and you need allow only an hour or two before switching to another medicine if there is no change. Wait twelve to twenty-four hours before you give a different medicine if symptoms are mild.

The symptoms of *Arsenicum* match those of many acute gastrointestinal affections. The classic patient has violent vomiting and diarrhea that can be accompanied by a great deal of pain in the stomach or intestines. The general characteristics determine the choice of this medicine: The patient is quickly exhausted by the illness, greatly weakened yet extremely restless; she constantly changes position until the weakness becomes completely debilitating. She may be very fearful and specifically afraid to be alone. The *Arsenicum* adult or older child often fears she has a serious illness and may die. There is usually a marked thirst; sometimes she repeatedly wants to drink small amounts of water. There may be a high fever, but the *Arsenicum* patient is typically very chilly and wants to stay under the blankets. When this combination of restlessness, exhaustion, fear, chilliness, and thirst is present during an acute digestive illness you should give *Arsenicum* no matter what the specific digestive symptoms.

The gastrointestinal symptoms of *Arsenicum* include severe nausea, vomiting, diarrhea, and abdominal pain. The symptoms come on or are worse at night, often after midnight. Vomiting is made worse by eating and drinking, and drinking even very little may cause immediate vomiting. Moving around or drinking milk may also result in renewed vomiting. Typically there is burning or cramping in the stomach or abdomen. In spite of the terrible burning, cold drinks aggravate the pain and warm drinks help. External warmth is also likely to help relieve the pain, whereas the patient's becoming chilled makes it worse. The diarrhea is also made worse by eating or drinking, particularly eating cold food, like ice cream, or drinking cold liquids. Burning may be felt in the rectum during or after the bowel movement. Great exhaustion follows. *Arsenicum* is the most commonly indicated medicine for food-poisoning illnesses.

Ipecac is indicated chiefly by persistent and extreme nausea, whether or not other symptoms such as vomiting or diarrhea are present. Even after vomiting, when most people would get at least temporary relief, the *Ipecac* patient may continue to feel sick to his stomach. The patient is usually not so severely ill in general as the *Arsenicum* patient, though he can certainly have a fever and feel weak. The nausea is made worse by the smell of food, and the condition can sometimes be traced to having eaten too much rich or fatty food. Most often there is a great deal of vomiting, sometimes becoming nearly continuous. Vomiting is worse after eating or drinking. Usually the person has little thirst and is not particularly anxious or chilly. The vomited material often contains much mucus. Pinching, cutting pains may be felt in the abdomen, and the persons often must pass much gas. Diarrhea accompanied by nausea is also a symptom of *Ipecac*. Stools are green, sometimes as green as grass, or frothy like yeast; they are often mucous. The tongue is usually clean and uncoated, and there is often increased salivating and drooling.

Colocynthis is indicated when the person complains of cramping, clutching abdominal pains that can be relieved with pressure and warmth. The patient may double up with the pain or he may press his fist into the painful area or lie over a hard object to get relief. Infants with *Colocynthis* colic are better when lying on the stomach but worse again if they are moved from that position. Warmth brings relief as well. The pain is made worse by eating and particularly by drinking. When the pain becomes severe enough, vomiting may occur; it often seems related to the intensity of the pain. Diarrhea may occur, with the stool preceded by the cramping pains described above. The bowel movement usually relieves the pain, at least for a time. Whatever the combination, the symptoms may have been brought on by the person's anger or suffering of an insult to his sense of justice.

Similarly, *Magnesia phos.* is useful to those with abdominal pain made better by warmth and pressure. If the two medicines can be distinguished, the *Magnesia phos.* patient finds greater relief in warmth and doesn't seek pressure so insistently. Vomiting and diarrhea are rare.

As always, *Belladonna* is indicated in the early stages of the illness if the symptoms came on suddenly. Gastrointestinal ailments' accompanying general symptoms—fever, flushed face, and dullness—are often as prominent as the nausea, vomiting, or diarrhea. Vomiting is not clearly related to eating or drinking; the vomited material contains mucus or partly digested food. *Belladonna* is likely to be helpful when infection elsewhere in the body comes on with vomiting or diarrhea in addition to the fever. There may be diarrhea with mucous stools. *Belladonna* also covers abdominal pains that are sharp and come on in spells, appearing and disappearing suddenly. The pains are worse after drinking and worsened by motion, being jarred, walking, or standing. Gentle pressure aggravates it, whereas firm pressure brings relief.

Bryonia is often the remedy for acute gastroenteritis. The general characteristic of this medicine, aggravation caused by motion, applies to all the digestive symptoms—nausea, vomiting, diarrhea, and abdominal pain may all be touched off by the slightest motion. Sometimes even moving a single part of the body is enough to bring on the symptoms. Vomiting comes on after eating or drinking. The smallest quantity of liquid may cause vomiting, though in some cases nausea is relieved by drinking. Abdominal pain is often relieved by pressure or by lying on the painful area, and it may improve after a bowel movement. Diarrhea is worse in the morning, after the patient gets up and moves around, and sometimes during hot weather. The stool is most often pasty or mushy. In general, the person feels warm, is irritiable, and wants to be left alone to lie still.

Phosphorus also covers certain symptoms of acute gastroenteritis. The symptoms are similar to those of *Arsenicum:* much vomiting and diarrhea, burning pains, weakness, anxiety and restlessness, and thirst for cold drinks. Usually, *Arsenicum* is a better first choice when these are the main symptoms, unless specific *Phosphorus* symptoms are present. Nausea is worse after warm drinks or even after putting the hands in warm water. Vomiting after eating or drinking is typical, but more specifically, the *Phosphorus* patient may vomit as soon as water becomes warm in the stomach or after drinking the smallest quantity of liquid. Warm water aggravates the vomiting immediately, and looking at water may cause renewed vomiting. Cold water momentarily relieves nausea and pain, but within a few moments it becomes heated and the symptoms begin again. There is often a general sense of emptiness and weakness in the stomach or entire abdomen, and an empty, hungry feeling may keep the person awake at night. The *Phosphorus* patient may experience diarrhea with involuntary stools. Sometimes the anus will not close and stool oozes out uncontrollably, or there may be only a sensation of an open anus.

Violent diarrhea, usually accompanied by vomiting, may best be covered by *Veratrum album*. The stools may look like water used to cook rice, or they may look watery and greenish, containing small green flakes. The stool is ejected forcefully from the body (more so than in the *Arsenicum* case) in great quantity. These symptoms are always accompanied by colicky cramps in the abdomen, which are temporarily relieved by the diarrhea. Violent vomiting is often associated with the diarrhea, and the person may purge from both the mouth and the rectum at the same time. Motion brings on renewed diarrhea and vomiting. The general symptoms of this medicine are marked and include severe chilliness, cold perspiration (especially on the forehead), and great weakness. The body is cold and even the breath may be cold. There is much thirst for large quantities of cold water.

Podophyllum is one of the most commonly indicated medicines for those with acute diarrhea. Profuse, offensive-smelling stools are characteristic. You may wonder where it all comes from since so much passes with each bowel movement and the movements are so frequent. The stools may be yellowish or greenish and are often completely liquid. The diarrhea is made worse by eating, drinking, and moving around, and it sometimes alternates with a headache. This medicine is well suited to the person with common diarrhea when he is a bit less energetic but not terribly sick; diarrhea seems to be the main symptom. Eventually, after frequent, profuse stools, he does become exhausted. *Podophyllum* diarrhea may be completely painless, or there may be abdominal pain that is worst before or during the bowel movement. Sometimes cramps in the muscles of the feet, calves, and thighs accompany the diarrhea, or yawning and stretching may be noticeable. Vomiting is rare, but dry heaves or gagging do occur at times.

When the symptoms have been brought on by mental exertion, overeating, or use of alcohol, coffee, or other drugs, *Nux vomica* can be a good medicine for those with gastrointestinal problems. Heartburn, nausea, empty retching, and sour burps are manifestations of a general disorder of the stomach. Headache, irritability, drowsiness, and dullness are typical of the *Nux* patient with digestive upset. The symptoms are worse in the morning and are also aggravated by eating; uncomfortable queasiness, bloating, and gas accumulation occur after meals. The patient often feels that this discomfort would be relieved if he could vomit, and vomiting after eating is common. This may take the form of retching up only small amounts of food. Vomiting or retching may follow his attempts to bring up phlegm from the throat. Diarrhea with brown liquid or mucous stools that come frequently in small amounts is characteristic. There may be a strong, sometimes constant, urge to move the bowels but little or no stool passes. A bad backache often precedes or accompanies the bowel movement. *Nux* matches the symptoms of many hangovers.

Pulsatilla also covers the digestive symptoms resulting from improper diet, in this case especially from rich foods, fats, or particularly ice cream. But *Pulsatilla* may benefit anyone with a

---

Beyond Home Care

These indications are for vomiting, diarrhea, indigestion, and abdominal pain.

Get Medical Care Immediately:

- for any severe abdominal pain;
- if there is incessant vomiting;
- if there is evidence of dehydration: lack of tears, truly dry mouth, loss of normal skin texture, sunken eyes, sunken soft spot in babies;
- if there is a possibility of poisoning or drug use;
- if vomited material or stools are bloody, black, red, tarlike, or resemble coffee grounds;
- if there is vomiting, diarrhea, or pain after an abdominal or head injury;
- if a child's vomiting is accompanied by marked irritability, inconsolable screaming, or marked lethargy.
- if vomiting begins unexpectedly during the course of a viral respiratory illness.

gastrointestinal condition if the general symptoms of the medicine are pronounced. Usually nausea, vomiting, and diarrhea are not too severe. There is heartburn, queasiness, a bad taste in the mouth, and a sense of heaviness after eating. The tongue may be coated thickly with white or yellow material. The person experiences nausea after drinking, especially drinking warm liquids, and cold drinks may relieve the nausea. Food eaten long before may be vomited up only partly digested. *Pulsatilla* also covers diarrhea with green or mucous stools or stools that constantly change in character or color. The diarrhea is likely to be worse at night, in a warm room, or when the patient gets warm.

Constipation

To stay in good health, it is not necessary to have a bowel movement every day, and no immediate health problems will result even if you go for a long time without one. Still, infrequent,

---

Get Medical Care Today:

- if there is significant vomiting or pain and no bowel movement for 24 hours;
- if the patient is or could possibly be pregnant;
- if the patient is diabetic;
- if there is yellowing of the skin or eyes, if the urine is very dark, or the stools are gray or nearly white;
- if there is swelling or pain in the groin or where the lower abdomen meets the thighs.

Call Your Practitioner Today:

- if you are taking any medications.

See Your Practitioner In the Next Few Days

- for recurrent abdominal pain, vomiting, or diarrhea, even if the symptoms are mild; or for any definite change in bowel habits lasting longer than two weeks.

difficult bowel movements are symptomatic of sluggishness of the intestines, which can contribute to cancer and diverticular disease and a variety of other degenerative diseases of the intestine, and possibly of the whole system.

General Home Care

The best way to alleviate constipation and maintain active bowel function is to drink adequate liquids and eat a diet rich in fiber. All plant foods contain a certain amount of indigestible "roughage." Since this material is not absorbed by the body, and in fact attracts and holds water, the stool is larger and stretches the intestinal walls. This stretching stimulates a reflex that speeds the movement of the stool through the intestine smoothly.

The foods richest in fiber content are whole grains and fresh vegetables; most fruits have less. You don't need to eat bran, the indigestible outer layer of grain, or to take any sort of laxative, as long as your diet includes plenty of whole grain and vegetables.

Sometimes these dietary measures fail to relieve constipation. At times an important factor may be stress of one kind or another, since the nervous system regulates the contraction of the intestinal muscles. Travelers commonly become constipated for this reason. A lack of exercise may also contribute to the problem.

Sometimes an internal imbalance is the real trouble, and no amount of dietary adjustment or stress reduction helps. Homeopathic treatment for people with chronic constipation can be helpful, but you should consult a professional if internal imbalance is suspected.

Beyond Home Care

Any time there is a marked change in bowel movement pattern that lasts more than a week or two, whether the new pattern develops slowly or gradually, you should consult your medical practitioner, especially if you are over thirty-five.

Hepatitis

Hepatitis, or inflammation of the liver, is most often caused by a viral infection. The most common hepatitis infections are hepatitis A, usually passed in the stool, and hepatitis B, passed mostly through blood or during sexual contact. Hepatitis B is more dangerous because a substantial proportion of those who come down with the disease develop chronic hepatitis, a serious chronic illness. Other viruses can cause hepatitis too, including mononucleosis. Sometimes poisons or drugs cause noninfectious hepatitis.

The symptoms of hepatitis include extreme fatigue, low-grade fever, disinterest in food, and queasiness. The liver may feel heavy, painful, and tender. *Jaundice,* a yellowing of the skin and eyes, sometimes but not always accompanies hepatitis. Likewise, very light-colored stools and very dark urine may or may not be noticed.

General Home Care

Hepatitis is a serious illness and you should have professional medical help to diagnose it and to follow its course. There are, however, no effective conventional medicines for hepatitis. Various preventive medications are available for people who have been or may in the future be exposed to hepatitis, and you should speak to your practitioner about them if you think you might be exposed.

If you have hepatitis, get as much rest as you feel you need, and eat a well-balanced diet of moderate protein and low fat content. Try to eat well even if you aren't very hungry. Avoid irritating spices, oily food, coffee, and drugs. You should entirely abstain from alcohol.

Homeopathic Medicines

Treatment with homeopathic medicines has often been successful in shortening the course of the illness and helping the person recover vitality. We have observed dramatic improvement in many cases. It is best to receive treatment from an experienced professional. If none are available, however, we think that you should treat yourself and your family. You should be receiving professional medical care whether or not you are using homeopathy at home.

Choose the medicine that seems to best cover the symptoms and give only three to six doses of it every twelve hours. Be sure to stop giving the medicine as soon as you notice any real change in the quality or intensity of the symptoms. If there has been no change within three or four days, try another remedy that fits the symptoms.

The earliest stage of acute liver disease sometimes calls for *Aconite* if the general symptoms of the remedy are also present— high fever, moaning, restlessness, and fearful anguish. Shooting pains in the region of the liver may be felt.

Belladonna may also be indicated for the person with hepatitis in the early stages, again, if the general characteristics of this medicine are evident. The pains in the liver come and go suddenly, and breathing, jarring motion, and lying on the right side worsen them.

Hepatitis with pain extending from the liver into the back and just below the right shoulder blade often indicates *Chelidonium*. The pains are sore or sticking in character, and eating may bring relief. From the region of the liver, they may radiate in any direction,

---

Beyond Home Care

Get Medical Care Today:

- if there is yellowing of the skin or eyes, if the urine is very dark, or if the stools are gray or whitish.

See Your Practitioner:

- if you think you have been exposed to hepatitis.
- if you have been experiencing unusual, unexplained fatigue or discomfort in the upper right part of the abdomen for more than a few days.

Consult the Beyond Home Care section on Abdominal Pain if the pain in the upper righthand quadrant is significant.

rather than just to the back. There is diarrhea with gray or yellow stools. The person feels heavy-headed and chilly, and there may be fever, jaundice, and a bitter taste in the mouth. The tongue may be coated yellow. There may be a craving for milk.

Lycopodium is an important medicine for people with hepatitis. The pains may extend into the back (as with *Chelidonium*), but they don't tend to be as sharp. There is likely to be a sense of being too full after only a few mouthfuls of food. Gas, bloating, and general abdominal discomfort develop immediately after eating, and there is often rumbling in the upper abdomen. The liver area can be sore to the touch and painful when lain upon, and the abdomen in general may be sensitive to the pressure of clothing.

The *Mercurius* hepatitis patient suffers from distressing symptoms of the upper digestive tract. The tongue may be coated a dirty yellow color, and it is likely to be swollen and puffy, taking the imprint of the teeth. The gums become swollen and weak and bleed easily. The liver is swollen and tender, and lying on the right side is painful. Stools may be light gray or yellowish green. The skin and eyes are often yellowed. There may be pronounced, clammy perspiration. A general sensitivity to both heat and cold is typical.

Nux vomica may be useful for the person with hepatitis, especially if she is a heavy alcohol or drug user. The accompanying symptoms may include those described earlier in this chapter. The liver may be swollen or sensitive to touch, and the pain is sometimes worse after mental work.

China suits the person with hepatitis when the liver is markedly sensitive to pressure and to touch. The patient is chilly and sensitive to open air. Like the *Nux* and *Lycopodium* patient, he may have a sense of heaviness or fullness in the stomach and abdomen, especially after eating. He may burp frequently, but this gives no relief. Burps taste bitter or like the food he has eaten. He may have cravings for cold drinks, sweets, or coffee.

Motion Sickness

Most people have been carsick or seasick at one time or another and know what an unpleasant experience it can be. If you are frequently bothered with the affliction of motion sickness, try one of these homeopathic medicines to prevent or treat the discomfort.

Cocculus covers the severe nausea, vomiting, and dizziness characteristic of motion sickness. Nausea and dizziness force the person to lie down; rising up, especially out of bed, and noise make them worse. The sight, smell, or even though of food brings on new waves of severe nausea. The symptoms are also worse when the throat is dry or when the patient gets cold.

The *Petroleum* patient gets dizzy and nauseated when riding in a car or boat. He becomes faint and pale and breaks out in a cold sweat. There may be pain in the back or the head, or there may be an empty, even painful sensation in the stomach that eating can relieve. He salivates excessively.

Tabacum symptoms include deathly nausea, possibly even worse than that of the other two medicines. The patient is cold and pale, and his body is bathed in cold perspiration. He suffers from violent vomiting with renewed retching every time he moves. His symptoms are particularly worse in warmth and are better in the open air, when the eyes are closed, and in a quiet, dark, environment. Occasionally he'll feel better after he uncovers the abdomen.

All of the above medicines are lesser-known homeopathic remedies and may be hard to come by. *Nux vomica* is a more commonly used medicine that also fits many of the symptoms of motion sickness. There is constant nausea, a splitting headache, and buzzing in the ears. More information on *Nux* appears earlier in this chapter and in the *materia medica*.

CHAPTER 9

Women's Health Problems

T HE women's medical self-care movement has probably done more to stimulate interest in self-care in general than
any other single factor. There are now many excellent books on
women's self-care, and many community clinics throughout the
country facilitate the learning of self-help skills and provide access
to health and medical information concerning the special health
needs and interests of women.

Homeopathic medicine offers a method of medicinal treatment
that complements other self-care measures for women's health
needs. Self-care with homeopathy can be very effective for some
simple women's problems, and in this chapter we will cover three
particularly common conditions: vaginal inflammation, menstrual
cramps, and cystitis. Women with many other gynecological problems can also be helped with homeopathy, but those with conditions such as irregular periods, abnormal menstrual bleeding,
ovarian cysts, uterine fibroids, breast conditions, sexual difficulties,
and so on should receive treatment from a professional homeopathic practitioner.

The homeopath values the symptoms of the reproductive system
as some of the most important clues about the well-being of the
whole person. The health of the reproductive system is a direct
reflection of the delicate balance and dynamic interplay between
two of the most central regulatory mechanisms of the body, the
hormonal and nervous systems.

Conventional medicine treats women's problems with drugs and
surgery that alleviate symptoms but do not remedy the underlying

disharmony. Even hormonal treatments commonly used by gynecologists: birth control pills, estrogens, progestins, and synthetic male hormones, work only for as long as they are taken and merely correct the levels of hormones circulating in the blood temporarily. They do not help the body regain the ability to self-regulate healthy hormone balance.

Obviously, homeopaths are wary of any such treatment that simply masks symptoms without restoring health. When the symptoms are no longer clearly apparent, important information about the nature of the woman's internal disorder is no longer available. More important, the body must compensate for the presence of the medicine in the system and for the changes in body chemistry it causes. Thus, the original imbalance is likely to be compounded and complicated by the treatment. Conventional treatment of some women's disorders, especially cancerous conditions, is certainly sometimes necessary. Whenever possible, however, we believe it is preferable to seek homeopathic care that encourages true healing before resorting to suppressive treatments.

Vaginitis

The lining of the vagina is a mucous membrane similar to the inside of the mouth. It is kept moist by secretions from cells in the membrane. The amount of fluid secreted by these cells changes in relation to the phase of the menstrual cycle and in response to sexual excitement. In addition, the cervix secretes liquid material that also varies in quantity and consistency during the menstrual cycle. Thus, the vagina normally contains small to moderate amounts of liquid. At certain times of the month the accumulation can be great enough to be noticed as a discharge, even when there is no infection or other problem with the vagina.

Abnormal discharge with vaginal inflammation or infection is termed *vaginitis*. There may be a substantial increase in the discharge; a change in its color, consistency, or odor; or accompanying symptoms such as itching or soreness. Sometimes the latter symptoms occur even though there is no appreciable discharge.

Prior to menopause the most common causes of vaginal inflammation are infections. Like the mouth and skin, the vagina is normally populated by a variety of microorganisms that serve to discourage infection. These "good" organisms control infectious germs by competing with them for food, by maintaining a chemical environment that inhibits their growth, and by forming a protective physical barrier. The vaginal lining also has a variety of immune defenses to further defend against infection. Women who have passed menopause or whose ovaries have been removed often experience vaginitis because of the reduced supply of hormones needed to maintain the vaginal tissues.

Vaginal infections begin when these normal protective mechanisms are disrupted by physiological imbalance, friction (as in vigorous sexual activity), drugs that kill the good organisms or alter hormone balance, or chemical irritation caused by diaphragm jelly or other products. Even wearing restrictive clothing or underwear made of synthetic materials may alter the vaginal environment enough to allow infection.

There are several common types of vaginitis. "Yeast," or *monilial,* infections are caused by the same fungal organism, *Candida albicans,* responsible for thrush in the mouth and for yeast rashes on the skin. This organism is actually a normal inhabitant of the human body and ordinarily lives in harmony with other microbes of the vagina. But when an imbalance occurs, the yeast invades the vaginal lining and reproduces rapidly. The infection, coupled with the body's reaction, produces the familiar symptoms of yeast vaginitis: thick, creamy or curdy, whitish discharge, often accompanied by itching or redness and rawness of the external genitals.

Bacterial infections of the vaginal lining are also common. The type of bacteria most frequently found in association with vaginal infections has been given various names (including *Hemophilus*), but is now called *Gardnerella.* Various other bacteria are sometimes found in association with vaginitis.

The third common cause of vaginal infection is the *Trichomonas* organism, an ameba-like microbe much larger than bacteria. *Trichomonas* infections typically result in a yellowish or greenish, sometimes frothy vaginal discharge. Often the cervix is involved in the infection and appears irregularly raw and reddened.

More serious infections of the female reproductive organs do occur. While less common than the three types of vaginal infection we've just mentioned, they are not at all rare. When bacteria such as *Gonococci* (gonorrhea), *Chlamydia,* and others infect the cervix, uterus, or fallopian tubes, there may be no symptoms at all. On the other hand, symptoms may range from vaginal discharge to inflammation of and pain in the internal organs, severe infection with pus formation, symptoms of general illness, and so forth. If untreated, these infections can result in infertility due to scarring within the fallopian tubes.

Vaginal inflammation and discharge can also occur without an infection or when infection plays only a minor role in causing the symptoms. Various kinds of irritating influences bring the body's local defenses into play to protect the tissues. The vaginal lining becomes red and swollen with extra blood, and secretions increase as an effort is made to flush the irritation away. Infection may result if the irritation allows germs to enter the tissues, but discomfort and a discharge don't necessarily mean an infection is present.

This type of noninfectious vaginitis may be caused by mechanical or chemical irritation due to vigorous sexual activity, by substances in diaphragm jelly, feminine hygiene products, tampons, or foreign objects in the vagina. Vaginal discharges that result from forgetting to remove a tampon are also fairly common.

General Home Care

If you're experiencing the early stages of mild vaginitis, you can certainly begin treatment at home. You don't have to know exactly what's causing the symptoms as long as you observe the guidelines in "Beyond Home Care." Even if you end up seeing your practitioner and perhaps receiving treatment, many of these self-care guidelines will probably apply.

First, consider whether or not there is something responsible for the vaginal-tissue irritation. Be sure you haven't left a tampon in place. If you've recently begun using a spermicidal jelly, contraceptive device, or vaginal deodorant, you may want to experiment with different brands or just avoid these things for a while to see if the irritation stops.

Remember to avoid synthetic fabrics in underwear, since these materials don't allow enough air to circulate. Loose-fitting clothing is preferable when possible.

Plenty of rest, limiting stress, and good nutrition often make the difference in how quickly and completely some women get over vaginitis. Diet has proven especially important to many women who have found that eating well-balanced meals and avoiding sweets in particular were helpful in preventing vaginal infections.

One of the specific measures most effective in helping heal vaginitis is using a vinegar douche, prepared by diluting two table-spoons of either white or apple cider vinegar in a pint of warm water, twice a day at first and then once a day as the symptoms improve. The healthy vagina is slightly acidic, and maintaining an acid pH by using vinegar helps promote the growth of the normal microorganisms that protect the lining and inhibit the growth of bacteria and *Trichonomas.* Yeast organisms prefer a more acidic environment, but vinegar has the specific ability to inhibit their growth. As with any douche, a vinegar douche cleanses the vagina of the overgrowth of infectious organisms.

Another treatment for vaginitis some women have found effective involves garlic. You can use garlic as a vaginal suppository by peeling off the clove's outer skin (while leaving the last thin layer of the skin intact) and inserting the clove into the vagina for twelve hours. Alternatively, you can place a crushed clove of garlic in vinegar and then, after straining the vinegar to remove the bits of garlic, use this liquid for a douche.

Trichomonas infections are particularly resistant to self-care measures. Some women have tried douching with strong chaparral tea (*Larrea divaricata*), though results have been inconsistent.

Medical treatments for common vaginal infections vary with the infectious organisms. Fungal infections are treated with antifungal suppositories or vaginal creams. Oral tetracycline is sometimes used to treat bacterial infection. Metronidazole (Flagyl) is an oral medication used for *Trichomonas* and bacterial infections.

Homeopathic Medicines

Home treatment with homeopathy is indicated if you have no major health conditions and if your symptoms are not recurrent. To use homeopathy for your vaginal infection, pay close attention to your symptoms before you use any douche or other treatment, since they determine the choice of the correct medicine. Pick the medicine that most closely matches your symptoms from the list that follows. Make certain to check with the *materia medica* section (part 4) for more details on the general symptoms of the leading homeopathic medicines. Take a dose one to three times a day, depending on severity, for up to three days. Stop as soon as your symptoms seem to be improving or changing substantially in any way. Allow two to three days without medicine before going on to another one if the first remedy doesn't seem to help.

Pulsatilla is useful to women with white vaginal discharges that have a consistency like milk or cream. Yellow discharges are also covered if the general symptoms suggest this medicine. The discharge may be either bland or irritating. It is one of the medicines appropriate for women with vaginitis during pregnancy (as are *Kreosote* and *Sepia*) or for pubescent girls (*Calcarea, Sepia*). Lying down may cause an increase in the discharge.

Calcarea Carbonica suits women with thick discharges that are either white or yellow. The discharge is likely to cause intense itching of the genitals. The flow of the discharge may come in sporadic gushes (*Graphites, Sepia*). This medicine may be indicated for young girls with vaginitis. Usually the choice of this medicine is confirmed by its general symptoms.

Graphites is indicated for women with thin, white, and burning discharges that tend to occur in large, periodic gushes. Weakness of the back or tension in the abdomen may accompany the vaginitis. Walking may increase the discharge, and it also may be worse in the morning (*Sepia, Kreosote*).

Sepia's most striking characteristic is a flow that is yellowish or greenish, but *Sepia* may suit women with almost any kind of flow. Offensive odor is typical of *Sepia* cases. The symptoms usually become worse shortly before the menses discharges or midway between them. As with *Graphites*, the *Sepia* discharge is likely to be more profuse in the morning and during walking. Sensations of uncomfortable pressure and weight ("bearing down pains") in the pelvic organs and lower abdomen are common in women who need *Sepia*. If no other symptoms suggest another medicine, give *Sepia* first when treating a child with vaginitis.

Kreosote is the first medicine to consider when the discharge causes or is associated with irritation and rawness of the vagina and external genitals, though other remedies also cover this symptom. There is soreness, smarting, burning, and itching in the tissues, and they become noticeably red and swollen with the inflammation. *Kreosote* discharges generally have a foul smell, which typically increases in the morning and upon standing.

Another important medicine indicated when the discharge is acrid, irritating, and offensive smelling is *Nitric Acid.* The *Nitric-Acid*-type discharge is greenish, brownish, flesh-colored, or sometimes like transparent, stringy mucus. Aggravation after the menstrual period is characteristic.

Borax is indicated when the vaginal discharge is clear and thick, like the white of an egg, or is thick and white, like liquid starch or sometimes even like white paste. The discharge may be bland or may irritate the genitals. A sensation of warmth may accompany the discharge, as if perhaps warm water were flowing over the organs. Sometimes the discharge is worst midway between the menstrual periods (*Calcarea, Kreosote, Sepia*). General symptoms of this medicine include a dread of downward motion and a marked sensitivity to sudden noises; however, these symptoms need not be present in every case.

Beyond Home Care

See "Beyond Home Care" that follows "Menstrual Cramps and Premenstrual Syndrome."

Menstrual Cramps and Premenstrual Syndrome (PMS)

Many women experience discomfort of one sort or another in association with their menstrual periods. Cyclic recurrences of symptoms such as uterine cramping, leg or back pain, nausea or diarrhea, bloating, swelling and tenderness of the breasts, irritability and depression, fatigue and listlessness, dizziness, rashes or pimples, and headaches may come before, during, or after the period, usually following a characteristic pattern for each woman.

There are many possible contributing causes for menstrual discomfort. Regulation of the phases of the menstrual cycle involves an intricate balance of complex physiological functions. There are cyclic variations in hormone levels, blood flow, nervous system function, prostaglandin levels, and so forth. Any imbalance may result in disordered menstrual function.

Unresolved emotional conflict may predispose some women to menstrual difficulties, acute or chronic. In other women, structural changes in the reproductive tract such as development of uterine fibroids or endometriosis make the menses painful. Lately, substances in the body called *prostaglandins* have been blamed for much of the trouble with difficult periods, but the prostaglandin disorder is really a *symptom* of a deeper imbalance.

General Home Care

Reducing stress levels may help prevent menstrual discomfort. Once you have cramps or other symptoms, you should certainly rest and take it easy as much as possible. Heat may bring some relief. Many women find that exercise during menstrual cramps also helps. Attention to general good nutrition can help minimize menstrual problems. In addition, some women have found that specific dietary measures including limiting intake of salt and dairy products reduce symptoms of PMS. Calcium and magnesium supplements may help as well; recommended amounts and proportion of these two nutrients depend on the individual's symptoms.

Homeopathic Medicines

Though symptoms may be relieved by taking medicines that, for example, block the action of prostaglandin, menstrual problems are not caused by simply one chemical abnormality that can be "fine-tuned" at will with drugs. In contrast, homeopathic constitutional treatment can catalyze a response of the entire system so that a better overall balance is achieved.

Recurrent menstrual cramps and other chronic difficulties associated with periods are best treated constitutionally. In some cases, even symptoms that are blamed on structural abnormalities are resolved with homeopathic treatment.

If constitutional care is not available, it is certainly acceptable to use homeopathic self-care when symptoms are acute. If you are already under constitutional treatment, however, you should not take homeopathic medicine without first consulting your homeopath.

Choose a medicine from among the following listed, and take it only during acute menstrual discomfort. You may repeat the medicine up to every four hours or so, but only if the symptoms have returned. Switch to a new medicine if you find no relief after eight to twelve hours.

Belladonna is commonly indicated for women suffering acute pain with their periods. The pains tend to begin suddenly and end just as suddenly. They may take the form of cramps or something like labor pains. There may also be a feeling of intense weight and pressure in the lower abdomen and pelvis, sometimes as though the pelvic organs were about to fall out. *Belladonna* patients with these bearing-down pains get relief by applying pressure to the genitals or abdomen. No matter what type of pain the woman has, *Belladonna* is indicated when motion, walking, or being jarred worsen it. Sitting bent over aggravates the pain, whereas straightening up makes it better. Pain may extend from the region of the uterus to the back. Pain in the ovaries before or during the menstrual period (again, if it is made worse by motion or jarring) is also typical of *Belladonna*. Headaches before and during the menses discharges are common (see chapter 11 on headaches).

If you have menstrual cramps that are unaccompanied by other symptoms and are relieved by pressure or warmth, either *Magnesia phos.* or *Colocynthis* is your choice. *Magnesia phos.* may bring relief if your menstrual pains are cramping in character or feel like the pains of childbirth, and if they are relieved by pressure, warmth, and bending forward. The pain centered in the uterus may radiate in all directions.

Colocynthis has nearly identical indications, with the pain being relieved by doubling up, pressure and warmth. *Colocynthis* pains are slightly more likely to make you double up. *Colocynthis* also covers sharp pains in the ovaries, especially when they occur shortly before the period. The *Colocynthis* patient is more likely to be irritable or angry than the woman who needs *Magnesia phos.* The cramps may have begun after the patient became angry or after she suppressed angry feelings.

Cimicfuga covers menstrual cramps that make the patient double over with pain. The particular indications for this medicine are sharp pains that dart from side to side in the abdomen and marked lower-back pain during the flow. Motion aggravates the pain.

Chamomilla is used for menstrual distress, as it is with other conditions, largely on the basis of the patient's mood. Marked irritability—faultfinding and snapping over little things—is typical. The menstrual pains are felt so acutely they may cause the woman to cry out. They may feel like cramps or labor pains (many remedies cover menstrual cramps that feel like labor pains, but *Chamomilla* fits this symptom better than any other homeopathic medicine). Sensations of weight and bearing down may also occur in the pelvis. Sometimes the pains seem to develop after getting angry. They are relieved by warmth.

Beyond Home Care

Get Medical Care Immediately:

- if there is severe pain (other than menstrual cramps) in the pelvic organs or abdomen.

Get Medical Care Today:

- if there is significant lower abdominal pain (not menstrual cramps), especially when accompanied by fever or vaginal discharge or bleeding. See the section on abdominal pain in chapter 8 on digestive problems;
- if there is vaginal discharge with lower abdominal pain or fever, or if it comes after you or a partner have had recent new sexual contact;
- if a girl develops a profuse vaginal discharge or irritation before puberty;
- if there are sores on or in the genitals or nearby areas, unless they are definitely recurrences of previously diagnosed herpes, *or* if there are *any* shallow open sores anywhere on the body that are not wounds;

The woman who needs *Pulsatilla* may also be irritable during her period, but not with the same angry intensity the *Chamomilla* patient has. She is sensitive, moody, weepy, or depressed, and perhaps a bit touchy, but she wants and appreciates gentle comforting. The menstrual pains may be of nearly any type and may be at their worst before or during the flow. They are sometimes bad enough to cause the woman to cry out or moan. Many other symptoms associated with periods may occur. Dizziness, fainting, nausea, vomiting, diarrhea, back pain, and headaches preceding or accompanying menstruation are all covered by *Pulsatilla*. Also, the woman has no thirst; heat worsens her condition, and open air makes it better.

The strongest indication for the self-care use of *Lachesis* is the symptom's being relieved when the menstrual flow begins. This

---

- if you have had sexual contact with someone known to have or suspected of having gonorrhea, syphilis, a *Chlamydia* infection, or any other major sexually transmitted disease. You don't need to be checked if you've simply been exposed to herpes or genital warts—wait to see if you develop symptoms;
- if there is heavy vaginal bleeding, even without pain, between the menstrual periods. Mild bleeding between the periods is common and is not a danger sign, unless it is persistent or recurrent.

See Your Practitioner Soon:

- if there has been persistent or recurrent, painless vaginal bleeding between the periods. If the bleeding lasts longer than ten days or recurs more than three months in a row, you need medical attention. If there is pain with the bleeding, seek care *now;*
- if there has been heavy vaginal discharge or significant genital irritation, or if a mild vaginal discharge lasts longer than two weeks;
- if there has been unusually heavy menstrual bleeding every month, or if you have severe menstrual cramps recurrently.

keynote characteristic pertains to any of the various symptoms that *Lachesis* suits: uterine pains, ovarian pain (especially on the left side), back pain, dizziness, headaches, and diarrhea, all of which may be severe before the period and then suddenly better once menstruation actually starts. Uterine cramps or soreness is likely to be made worse when clothing contacts the abdomen, especially tight belts or elastic bands. The pains may extend into the upper abdomen or chest. Classic *Lachesis* symptoms begin or worsen during sleep or immediately upon wakening.

Caulophyllum should be considered when cramping pains are particularly bad before the period starts, though there is less immediate relief from the onset of the flow than with *Lachesis*. Pain in the small of the back or dizziness may also precede menstruation.

Cystitis

Fifteen percent of all adult women get repeated bladder infections. The common symptoms of *cystitis*, or bladder infection, include a burning pain during urination, a frequent and powerful urge to urinate though little urine may be passed, and cloudy or bloody urine. Pain or tenderness in the lower abdomen or the back, fever, and a feeling of being generally ill may also accompany cystitis.

The reasons women are so susceptible to urinary infections are that the *urethra,* the tube connecting the bladder to the outside of the body, is only one-half inch long and that the opening of the urethra is close to the anus. Bacteria from the intestinal tract can easily travel to the urethra and then into the bladder, where they can infect susceptible tissues. Bladder infections are more likely to occur after sexual activity or improper hygiene that allows germs to spread to the urethra. Anything that irritates the urethral tissue, such as an improperly fitted diaphragm, spermicidal jelly, or tight-fitting clothing, may weaken resistance to infection. Urinary tract infections are also more frequent during pregnancy.

As long as the infection is confined to the urethra and bladder, an attack of cystitis may be uncomfortable but not dangerous. What poses the real threat is the infection's spreading into the kidneys. Kidney infection can be a serious illness with its high fever, marked weakness, and back pain. But of greater concern is that inflammation occuring during a kidney infection can result in permanent damage to the kidneys.

Conventional medical treatment for urinary tract infections involves antibiotics, which usually soon control the acute infections but do nothing to prevent further bouts. During a bladder infection, you should be under the care of your health professional, though you may not need to take antibiotics immediately if you follow the self-care guidelines carefully and take an appropriate homeopathic medicine.

Some women experience the symptoms of cystitis but do not have a bacterial infection. Antibiotics are of no value in these cases.

General Home Treatment

Many urinary infections can be prevented by simple self-care measures. Hygiene is important. Always wipe from front to back after using the toilet, and be sure to change tampons or sanitary napkins frequently during menstruation. Drink lots of fluids and urinate often, at least every two hours, to help wash germs out of the urethra. Urinating as soon as possible after lovemaking is especially important. Avoid potential irritants such as deodorant tampons, "feminine hygiene" products, and strong or perfumed soaps. Use cotton rather than synthetic-fabric underwear. Avoid caffeine, which may irritate the urinary tract's tissues. Diaphragms should be fitted properly to prevent pressure on the urethra. If you use birth control pills, get a low- or no-estrogen kind.

If you do begin to have burning or frequent urination, you should immediately begin drinking more liquids to dilute the bacteria in the bladder and flush them out. Making the urine more acidic by drinking plenty of unsweetened cranberry juice or by taking vitamin C (be sure you take the ascorbic acid form, not ascorbate) helps slow down the reproduction of the bacteria.

Homeopathic Medicines

Select a medicine from the list below and give a dose every six to eight hours for up to two days, stopping as soon as the symptoms significantly change. Go on to another medicine if the symptoms are no better after twenty-four hours.

As with many inflammatory conditions, *Aconite* should be considered during the earliest stages. The patient may notice at first that it is difficult to pass urine, and then begins to experience burning pain during urination. At the same time, the general symptoms of *Aconite* may be developing.

Cantharis is the most commonly effective homeopathic medicine in treating those with urinary tract infections. Patients who need

Beyond Home Care

Get Medical Care Today:

- in general, whenever there is onset of acute urinary symptoms: burning pain in the urinary passageway, frequent or strong urges to urinate, or definitely cloudy urine. You may postpone medical care for forty-eight hours if pain is slight, frequency is mild, and there are no other symptoms;
- if the patient who has urinary pain or who must urinate frequently is a diabetic or has a history of high blood pressure or kidney disease;
- if the patient is a child who has urinary pain or must urinate frequently;
- if there is blood in the urine (the urine may look smoky red or brown);
- if there is headache, vomiting, back pain, muscular twitching, convulsions, or chills along with urinary tract pain;
- if there are sharp pains in the kidney area, located in the back above the lower ribs;
- if a fever accompanies urinary pain;
- if there is any swelling of the face, ankles, or abdomen;

See Your Practitioner Soon:

- if there are any recurrent urinary symptoms;
- if there is significant weight loss.

(If there is a vaginal discharge, consult the "Beyond Home Care" section for vaginitis.)

Cantharis have a frequent, strong urge to urinate, and a great deal of burning is felt during urination. The patient may be compelled to rush to the toilet, and the urgency may be such that she loses urine before she gets there. Despite the intolerable urging, however, urine may pass in drops only. Strong urging may be felt immediately after voiding or even during urination itself. Tremendous burning, cutting, or stabbing pains are felt in the urethra and bladder before, during and after urination, or whenever the urge to urinate is felt. The patient is restless, even frantic, with the severe pain. Sexual desire may be increased.

Sarsaparilla should be considered when the most severe pain in the urethra comes at the end of urination. It may not be burning in character. The bladder is less likely to be painful than it is in the *Cantharis* or *Nux* patient. Sometimes the patient can only urinate in dribbles while sitting down and must stand up to get urine to flow freely.

Mercurius may be indicated during a bladder infection if the symptoms are worse at night, or if the general symptoms of the medicine are clearly present. All the typical symptoms of cystitis are covered by *Mercurius,* including burning, uncontrollable urges, dark urine, and passage of urine in small amounts. *Mercurius* is one of the few medicines indicated when burning pain is worse when the patient is not urinating; burning may be also severe just before urination, upon beginning to urinate, or when the last drops are passed.

The *Nux vomica* patient may also suffer the typical symptoms of bladder infection and may be given *Nux* on the basis of its general characteristics. Distinguishing urinary symptoms of *Nux* include burning or pressing pain in the bladder during urination, pain in the urethra before or during urination (sometimes accompanied by a strong urge to have a bowel movement), and needlelike pains in the urethra extending back toward the bladder. The woman may experience her urinary symptoms after excesses in eating, alcohol, coffee, or drugs.

Berberis should be considered when there are pains during or after urination, cutting or shooting either from the bladder to the urethra or from the urethra to the pelvis, thighs, or back. Motion may bring on pain. The patient may also experience pain in the area of the ureters or kidneys that worsens with pressure, motion, or jarring.

Pulsatilla is most often used to treat women who have cystitis as well as the classic *Pulsatilla* disposition. Although the pain may not be quite as intense as that of the *Cantharis* patient, there is significant smarting and burning. Lying on the back may aggravate the urging enough to rouse the patient from sleep if she turns from her side onto her back. Urine may pass only in dribbles, and there may be involuntary dribbling at the slightest provocation, including coughing, sneezing, laughing, or being surprised.

Apis should be considered in treating people who have cystitis with severe pain and urging similar to those described for *Cantharis*. The burning and especially stinging pains are worse in the heat and at night and better in cold. Though there is violent urging, the patient must strain to urinate, and the urine passes only in drops. The abdomen is sensitive to the slightest touch.

CHAPTER 10

Men's Health Problems

The health of the male reproductive system is a reflection of overall well-being as well as sexual habits. We cover common men's health concerns, including urethritis, venereal diseases, prostate problems, irritation of the foreskin, and briefly, less common serious problems of the testicles.

Urethritis and Venereal Diseases

The modern term for venereal disease is "sexually transmitted disease," or STD. There are about fifteen of these infectious illnesses that may be transmitted during lovemaking. Symptoms of these infections include various kinds of eruption and soreness on the genitals or surrounding skin and swelling of the lymph nodes in the groin. Most of these illnesses require medical treatment. Two common, but not very serious, sexually transmitted illnesses are genital herpes simplex and venereal warts, both of which are discussed in chapter 13 on skin problems.

Urethritis is infection and inflammation of the lining of the urethra, the tube that runs the length of the penis, carrying urine and semen. Urethritis is most often associated with sexually transmitted infections, though sometimes no infection can be documented. A variety of germs can infect the urethra and trigger the body's inflammatory response, which can result in symptoms of burning and stinging as well as discharge of mucus or pus.

Unlike women, males rarely get bladder infections, mostly because the urethra is longer and not so near the anus. A bladder infection in a boy or man is often evidence that something is structurally wrong with the urinary organs, and he must be evaluated by a urologist.

Though gonorrhea is the most notorious cause of male urethritis, urethral infections are more frequently caused by the *Chlamydia* bacteria. Before this bacteria was identified, physicians had described any case of urethritis not caused by gonorrhea as "nonspecific urethritis." Occasionally this infection can lead to chronic problems in men, and it is often passed on to women, possibly causing infections of the female reproductive tract, resulting in pain, illness, and sterility. There are many other kinds of germs less commonly associated with urethritis in men. Most of these are not now considered causes of health problems, but they have not been well studied. Urethritis can sometimes be caused by irritation, or it may occur after taking antibiotics.

The most worrisome infection of the urethra is gonorrhea, since the gonorrhea bacteria can spread to other parts of the body, causing general illness and infections in the large joints—usually elbows and knees—and since it, again, can cause serious infections in women. A gonorrhea infection of the urethra usually causes the penis to discharge a copious, thick, yellowish pus, along with burning pain at the opening of the urethra, felt during urination especially. In some cases, however, the discharge may be watery, scanty, or completely nonexistent, and there may be no pain. Gonorrhea can also infect other mucous membranes. Gonorrhea infections of the throat and rectum after oral or anal sex are not uncommon. Rectal gonorrhea may result in pain or discharge of pus, or there may be no symptoms at all.

We want to point out once again that the symptoms of all urethral infections, even when caused by gonorrhea, are largely evidence of the body's efforts to heal and remove the aggressive germs. Inflammation brings blood to the area so that more white blood cells, antibodies, and other components of the body's immune system are available to help destroy the bacteria. The extra blood also helps carry away dead cells and speeds the replacing of tissue damaged by the infection. The discharge flushes away debris and dead bacteria and blood cells, as well as much of the infecting germs.

Still, we strongly recommend antibiotic treatment, along with homeopathic treatment, for anyone with gonorrhea or *Chlamydia* urethral infections.

Discharges are uncommon in children but may develop if a child has put something in the urethra. A child with a penile discharge needs medical care.

General Home Care

Home treatment of urethritis should be begun whether or not you ultimately take antibiotics. Drink extra fluids and urinate frequently to wash the germs out of the urethra. You should pay attention to the general health practices of resting, eating a simple and nutritious diet, and avoiding stress, for these enable the body's own defenses to better fight the germs and heal the inflamed tissue.

Homeopathic Medicines

Homeopathic medicines should also be used, particularly if it is determined that antibiotics are not necessary, or if you continue to have symptoms after you've completed antibiotic treatment. Take a dose of the medicine you choose from the following list twice a day for two or three days; stop as soon as symptoms improve. Unless there is marked pain, allow a day or two without taking anything before you try another medicine.

Natrum muriaticum is one of the primary medicines for men with urethritis. The discharge is usually thin and clear, mucous, or milky in color. Sometimes a greenish discharge occurs. The discharge may appear clear when it is wet but then leaves yellow spots on the underwear. There may be cutting or burning pains at the urethral opening during or after urination or just as urination is finished.

Pulsatilla should help men with thick, yellow or green urethral discharge that is bland and causes little pain. The medicine's general symptoms may indicate its use more than the specific symptoms of the discharge.

Mercurius is indicated when thick mucus or pus is accompanied by inflammation and burning pain of the urethra. The discharge may be white, yellow, or green. Often the symptoms are worse at night.

Sulphur should be considered for thin or mucous discharges when there is burning pain during ejaculation or when the general symptoms of the medicine are evident. *Nitric Acid* is also a possibility when the discharge is accompanied by burning pain during ejaculation. The discharge is more likely to be thick and greenish or yellowish. The urine may smell very strong. The patient is usually chilly.

Prostatitis

The walnut-size prostate is located at the floor of the pelvis behind the base of the penis. During ejaculation the prostate contributes a milky alkaline fluid to the semen to enhance the fertility of the sperm.

Because the urethra passes through the prostate on its way from the bladder, bacteria can travel through the urethra to settle in the prostate. The prostate gland is susceptible to both acute infection and to chronic infection or inflammation. An acute infection can cause severe pain and tenderness in the region of the prostate, sometimes extending up into the genitals, pelvis, or back; acute infection can cause increased urge to urinate, burning during urination, difficulty starting urination, penile discharge, and general symptoms such as fever and weakness.

Chronic inflammation of the prostate can develop after an acute infection or on its own. Symptoms are similar to but milder than those of acute infection and tend to come and go over long periods. Vague aching in the region of the prostate, dribbling of urine, trouble starting or maintaining a forceful stream of urine, and discharge of prostatic fluid from the penis after a bowel movement, for instance, are common symptoms. Often it is impossible to identify the bacteria involved in chronic prostatitis; it may well be a self-perpetuating problem that persists even after infecting bacteria have been eliminated.

The prostate grows larger with age. It is common for late-middle-aged and older men to have problems urinating, because swelling of the prostate gland constricts the urinary passage. There may be trouble getting the urinary stream started, or the stream may be weak or interrupted. Frequent urging to urinate, together with passing of only small amounts, is common. These symptoms should be evaluated medically.

General Home Care

Home treatment for acute prostatitis includes drinking plenty of fluids, urinating frequently to help wash out the infecting bacteria, getting rest, eating a simple, nutritious diet, and avoiding stress to help the body heal.

Chronic prostatitis is difficult to heal completely. If the fluid made and stored by the prostate is allowed to accumulate, it can put pressure on the tissues and harmfully increase the inflammation. The prostatic fluid also serves as a growth medium for the bacteria infecting the gland. Therefore, it is a good idea for men with chronic prostatitis to ejaculate regularly, once every one or two days, in order to keep the prostatic fluid from building up. The home treatment described for men with acute prostatitis is applicable here as well.

Prostatic massage helps to empty the prostate gland more completely and is often used by health practitioners in the treatment of chronic prostatitis. A milder form of self-massaging the prostate some have tried is Kegel exercises: firmly tighten the muscles you would use to interrupt the flow of urine and repeat 50 to 100 times per day.

Homeopathic Medicines

During either acute or chronic prostatitis, homeopathic home care may be a reasonable alternative to conventional antibiotics if they don't work very well and the responsible bacteria are not dangerous. We recommend you see an experienced, professional homeopath if one is available, but if not you may go ahead and try one of these medicines.

During acute symptoms, give a dose two to three times a day for up to four days. Stop as soon as the symptoms improve, and repeat the dose thereafter only if they are definitely worse again. Switch to another medicine if there is no improvement after thirty-six to forty-eight hours. If prostatitis is chronic, use only a single dose of the medicine a day for five days. Wait at least two weeks before changing to another medicine.

Pulsatilla is a good medicine for the man who experiences aggravation of pain in the prostate after urination. There may be sharp pains or spasms in the region of the prostate that extend into the bladder and pelvis. There may be a thick, bland discharge from the penis. Men who show strong general symptoms of this medicine can be given *Pulsatilla* even when the specific symptoms don't clearly confirm it.

Chimaphilla umbellata is more difficult to find—even at a homeopathic pharmacy—than most of the medicines covered here, but it is well indicated for many men with prostatitis. Soreness in the region of the gland is worse with pressure, especially during sitting. There may be a sensation of sitting on a ball or simply of painful swelling. A discharge of mucus from the penis or the presence of stringy mucus in the urine may be noted.

The *Kali bichromium* patient's prostate pain is worsened by walking, and he must stand still for relief. The pain may be needlelike or there may be drawing pains extending from the prostate into the penis. There may be burning in the urethra after urination. A discharge of particularly thick, sticky, or stringy material may be found at the urethral opening.

The pains the *Apis* patient has are stinging in character. They may involve the bladder as well as the prostate, and they are worse during urination.

With *Causticum* there are pressure and pulsations in the prostate with pain extending into the urethra and bladder after a few drops of urine have passed. In contrast, *Lycopodium* covers pressure in the gland that is worse during and after urination, possibly with needlelike pains in the bladder and anus.

Foreskin Irritation

If a skin irritation on or under the foreskin develops, you can treat it at home by gently pulling the foreskin back, applying dilute *Calendula tincture* (see chapter 14), and allowing the area

Beyond Home Care

Get Medical Care Immediately:

- if there is significant pain in the testicles;
- if you pull the foreskin back and cannot return it to its normal position.

Get Medical Care Today:

- for babies, if the opening of the foreskin is too small to allow urine to pass freely;
- if there is swelling or lumps within a testicle;
- if there is a sore on the genitals or nearby areas, unless you are sure it is a recurrence of previously diagnosed herpes. Sores caused by syphilis in particular can appear on the body, usually on the hands or in or around the mouth. If you develop an unexplained, shallow, open sore, whether or not it is painful, and if you or a partner have had new sexual contacts within the past two months, see your practitioner;
- if there is significant pain in the prostate region, particularly if there is also a fever or back or pelvic pain;
- if there is a discharge from the penis, particularly if you or a partner have had new sexual contacts within the last two weeks;
- if you have had sexual contact with someone known to have or suspected of having gonorrhea, syphilis, a *Chlamydia* infection, or any other major, sexually transmitted disease. You don't need to see your practitioner if you've simply been exposed to herpes, genital warts, or a yeast infection—wait to see if you get symptoms.

See Your Practitioner Soon:

- if you have had difficulty starting urination, trouble with a weak or interrupted urinary system, or dribbling of urine.

to dry before returning the foreskin to its normal position. If a sexually active adult has sores or a rash, or if pus has formed, see your practitioner.

Occasionally the foreskin may get stuck in a retracted position and may become swollen or inflamed. Apply ice wrapped in a cloth to the area and try to gently work the foreskin back into its normal position. If you are not immediately successful, emergency care is required.

Testicular Problems

Epididymitis is an infection of the *epididymis*, a compact, coiled tube attached to each testicle and in which newly formed sperm mature. Although epididymitis does not occur too often, it is more common than *orchitis*, infection of the testicles. Both these infections cause pain and swelling in the testicular area.

Testicular pain may also be caused by twisting of the testicle and the structures within the scrotum that connect it to the body. This is not only extremely painful but also dangerous, because if the blood supply is interrupted, the testicle may be lost in a few hours.

Testicular cancer is one of the most common cancers in men under thirty. You should get checked immediately if you notice change in the size of or any lumps or nodules in a testicle. Testicular cancer is usually easy to treat when it is discovered early. Men should make it a habit to regularly feel their testicles (in the shower is a good time) to be sure that no changes have occurred.

CHAPTER 11

Headaches

Most of us have one or two "weak links," that is, parts or systems of our bodies that are the first to show evidence of the struggle to cope with an overload of physical or psychological stress. Some people get colds, some digestive upsets, and a great number are prone to headaches. Headaches, in fact, account for more doctor's visits than any other single health condition.

Some people suffer from headaches that are severe or frequent enough to be literally incapacitating and certainly, there are times when a headache can be a signal that something serious is wrong. In the great majority of cases, however, the pain of a headache can best be seen as a message that the level of stress in a person's life has exceeded his body's ability to adapt to it smoothly and healthfully. The headache serves as a warning that you need a change, perhaps a rest, deal with an emotional conflict, change your diet, or reduce your exposure to a toxic substance.

Modern medicine classifies headaches according to the immediate cause of painful stimulation of nerve endings. The types of headaches include muscle-contraction headaches, vascular headaches, and headaches caused by inflammation or structural conditions.

Muscle-Contraction Headaches

Nearly everyone has had a *muscle-contraction headache,* more commonly but less precisely referred to as a "tension headache." Most people assume that the term "tension" refers to emotional stress, and in fact, many times this type of headache is brought on by encountering pressure on the job, being stuck in a traffic jam, or other such situations. But the pain of a muscle-contraction headache arises from tightening of the muscles of the upper back, neck, and scalp, and this may result from any type of stress, whether physical or emotional. Extremes of heat or cold, hunger, loss of sleep, a tiring drive, and improper posture are all examples of physical stresses that can lead to muscle-contraction headaches.

The body reacts to different types of stress in a variety of ways, including increasing muscle tone to prepare us to meet stressful situations. A headache occurs once a certain threshold of tension in the muscles of the head and neck is reached. The pain arises, partly because the muscle is simply sore from being overworked, and partly because the tension constricts blood vessels and reduces blood flow to the tiring muscles. It is now thought that many or most muscle-contraction headaches are accompanied by some degree of the physiological changes that account for vascular headaches (see the next section in this chapter).

The pain of a muscle-contraction headache is typically a dull, steady ache felt along the forehead, at the temples, or at the base of the head and neck. A sensation of tightness, as if a constricting band were wrapped around the head, may be felt. The scalp and neck are usually tender to the touch.

General Home Care

Muscle-contraction headaches are generally easy to treat at home: simply take a break from the stress that led to the headache, get some rest, and perhaps massage the sore neck muscles. If the headache doesn't respond to these simple measures within a short time, try a homeopathic medicine from the list in this chapter. By helping the body restore order and balance, the correct homeopathic medicine speeds relaxation of the muscle contraction and relief from the pain, without any of the side effects associated with aspirin or acetaminophen.

Steps you can take to prevent recurrent muscle-contraction headaches include:

1. Be sure that the cause of the muscle tension is not a simple physical one like poor posture, uncomfortable clothing, or envi-

ronmental conditions (too chilly, irritating noise, and so on). It may be helpful to keep a written record of your headaches and of the stresses you experience prior to their onset. Notice whether you have any habits that are awkward or cause tension and straining, such as the way you sit at your desk, hold the telephone, or clench your jaw. Sometimes massage or some of the specialty body-work practices—such as the Alexander technique, chiropractic, rolfing, or acupressure—are helpful in treating or preventing this type of headache. While it is not a common cause of headache, eyestrain due to poor eyesight is occasionally to blame.

A sometimes-neglected cause of muscle tension is misalignment of the temporomandibular joints (TMJ) just in front of the ears around the lower jaw. If your headache pain is relieved by placing a two-to-three inch piece of Popsicle stick or tongue depressor between the teeth to separate the upper and lower jaws, you may have a problem with TMJ. Evaluation of TMJ disorders is best performed by a specially trained dentist.

2. Recognize and deal with situations in your life that cause emotional stress.

3. Learn how to relax the muscles that tense up during a headache, and learn to set the threshold of your stress reaction a little higher. We suggest you set aside ten-minutes or so twice a day for relaxation exercises; try to relax your whole body and your head and neck muscles in particular. Biofeedback can help you learn to control various physiological processes that lead to tension headaches, as can meditation. Exercise and massage are both great for relieving tension and depression.

If you apply these relaxation methods to your daily life, your stress reaction will be triggered less easily. Spend the last few moments of each period of relaxation imagining yourself in the situation that causes you the most stress—perhaps it's driving in rush hour traffic—but keep that relaxed feeling. After a week or so, you'll start to remember the relaxation sessions whenever you're in that tense situation, and before long, you'll find that you can maintain greater tranquillity even then.

For more details on learning to deal with stress, see Pelletier's *Mind as Healer, Mind as Slayer* (1977) and Jaffe's *Healing from Within* (1981).

4. Learn to recognize the early signs and sensations of tension, both muscular and emotional. If you can sense tension before a

bad headache comes on, you can do something to break the cycle before tension increases. Get out of the stressful situation for a few minutes, do some physical exercise to help release stored tension, meditate, pray, or do anything you find relaxing or joyful (laughter is great for releasing tension).

5. Some people get muscle-contraction headaches when they are hungry or have eaten combinations of foods that are difficult to digest. Pay attention to the pattern of your headaches in relation to diet. We recommend regular meals with an emphasis on fresh vegetables, whole grains and, if desired, lean meats; also, avoid sweets and caffeine. Specific foods often aggravate vascular headaches, and since many headaches may be of mixed type, it may be useful to avoid these foods.

For more information on self-treatment of headaches, we recommend *The Woman's Holistic Headache Relief Book* by June Biermann and Barbara Toohey.

Vascular Headaches

Many people use the word "migraine" to refer to any really bad headache, but *migraine headache,* as medically understood, denotes that pain resulting from a complex series of specific changes in the blood vessels of the head and brain. During a migraine, the blood vessels first become overly constricted and then widen abnormally. This sequence of constriction–widening affects the blood vessels on one side of the head more intensely, and often it is especially pronounced in a particular area of the brain.

The symptoms of migraine headaches are directly related to these changes in the blood vessels. During the initial phase of blood vessel narrowing, decreased blood flow to the brain leads to malfunction in the area of greatest constriction. So, before any pain is felt, the typical migraine begins with some sort of warning symptom, called an aura. The most common aura is disturbance of vision, which may take the form of bright or colored zigzag lines, areas of cloudy vision, flashing lights, and so on. Other people have auras with such symptoms as slurred speech, dizziness, weakness or numbness of one side of the body, and other signs of neurological impairment.

The migraine headache pain begins when the previously narrowed blood vessels then open too wide. Normal brain function is restored by the return of blood flow, but stretching of the vessel walls, along with inflammation caused by chemical changes in the blood, stimulates pain-sensitive nerve endings in the vessel walls. At first the pain is localized on one side of the head, but it often spreads to the other side as the headache progresses. The pain is intense and throbbing in character. Accompanying the headache may be symptoms such as nausea, vomiting, or diarrhea; intolerance of light, dizziness; and sweating or chilliness.

This description of the migraine applies to the "classic" type, but other forms of migraine are not uncommon. Sometimes the headache begins without a prior aura. On the other hand, "migraine equivalents" may occur; there may be the neurological disturbances (visual changes and so on) or vomiting typical of a migraine, though there is no headache.

The tendency to have migraines clearly runs in families and seems to be due, in part, to a genetic predisposition. They first occur before the person reaches the age of thirty, usually in the early-teen years. Migraines often start in childhood, particularly around the time of puberty. Even very young children can get migraines. Before the child is old enough to tell you about the headache, the first sign you may see in your two-to-four year old is recurrent vomiting. The child who gets headaches may well be saying something about a difficulty in her life that she finds difficult to express openly. Do your best to identify stress your child faces, and work with her to find ways to resolve the conflict.

A migraine headache is most often triggered by psychological stress but, curiously, it is characteristic that the attack begin when the stress is relieved. High-pressure business people, for instance, may dread the "relaxing" weekends that bring on their headaches. Other stresses that frequently lead to migraines include going without food, sleeping too long, bright lights, and fluctuations in hormone levels (some women get migraines every month when they ovulate or during the menstrual period). Foods and drinks including nuts, chocolate, coffee, cheese, citrus, and alcohol may also trigger migraines, as do some drugs.

Another type of vascular headache is the "cluster headache." These are severe, one-sided headaches that occur in spells, most often during sleep. The pain is accompanied by redness and tearing of the eye, and the nostril drops on the painful side.

General Home Care

An untreated migraine lasts at least several hours, often a full day. Many migraine headaches are so severe, simple measures like rest or aspirin offer little or no help. Relaxation measures may bring some relief. Learning to warm the hands by increasing blood flow through biofeedback has been especially effective, probably because the circulatory system in general is affected. Suggesting to yourself that the hands are becoming warm and heavy is the best way for most people to achieve this without a biofeedback device.

Dealing effectively with stress and avoiding the factors that you know lead to your headaches are the best ways to prevent migraines. Constitutional homeopathic treatment from a professional practitioner is the most helpful preventive approach for those whose headaches don't respond to simple home care measures or to self-care homeopathy.

The conventional medicines used to treat and prevent migraines are strong drugs with many potentially serious side effects. We strongly recommend that they be used as a last resort and that you try self-care methods and homeopathic treatment first.

Other Headaches

Less common than muscle-contraction and migraine headaches are the various types of headaches caused by infection, inflammation, and structural changes in the face and head. Many of these are serious conditions requiring medical treatment.

For information about acute sinus headaches, see the section on sinus conditions in chapter 4 on colds and coughs.

Homeopathic Medicines for Headaches of All Types

Use homeopathic medicines at home when you or your children have mild-to-moderate headaches. Give a dose of the medicine up to every two hours. Once improvement has begun, repeat the dose only if the symptoms are definitely worse again or improvement has ceased for an hour or so. If you are no better after two or three doses of the first medicine you try, switch to the one that seems the next best match for the symptoms.

It can sometimes be difficult to choose the right homeopathic medicine for a headache. So many headaches are made better or worse by the same factors, many remedies cover these common modalities. Often the person's general symptoms are your best guide in choosing the medicine. Use only the strongest, most definite headache symptoms in your case analysis, and compare them to the symptoms we list here. If you still have trouble picking the right medicine, we recommend you choose between the first three we cover, *Belladonna*, *Nux*, and *Bryonia*, for one of these three medicines will help the majority who suffer from acute headaches that have few other symptoms.

Belladonna is indicated for people whose headaches are intense with violent throbbing pains. The headache causes an extreme sensitivity, and the least bit of light, noise, touch, strong or unusual smell, motion, or jarring brings on a new wave of throbbing and pain. The pain often begins suddenly, and it may go away suddenly as well. It may spread throughout the entire head, or it may be localized anywhere, but perhaps it is most typically focused in the forehead; from the forehead it may extend to the back of the head. Often the face is flushed or feels hot, and sometimes the hands and feet are cold. *Belladonna* is thus the most commonly given medicine for headaches associated with high fever. The pupils may be noticably dilated during a *Belladonna* headache.

Firm pressure applied to the head helps (other remedies have this modality). Lying down may relieve or aggravate it, but *Belladonna* is unique, as it suits headaches that are definitely relieved by sitting. *Belladonna* is one of a number of medicines that cover headaches made worse by climbing steps, but it alone fits those also aggravated by traveling down a slope or stairway. Afternoon is most characteristically the time of worst pain.

Bryonia is best used when the most prominent characteristic of the headache is aggravation with motion. Both *Belladonna* and *Bryonia* cover this marked sensitivity to motion, and many other remedies are made worse by motion to some degree, but for the *Bryonia* patient, it is the outstanding characteristic. Even slight motion of the head or eyes worsens the pain. The pain is made worse by slight touch but made better by firm pressure. It is generally worst in the morning, and though it may be felt immediately upon waking, it is just as likely to come on only after the person first moves in bed or after she gets out of bed. There is little throbbing with *Bryonia* headaches, unlike those of *Belladonna,* and the pain is described as a steady ache, sometimes with a sense of fullness or heaviness. As with *Belladonna,* the headache is likely to be located in the forehead, extending from there to the back of the head, but it is commonly centered over the left eye, a symptom not shared with *Belladonna.* Nausea, vomiting, and especially constipation may occur in connection with *Bryonia* headaches. The *Bryonia* patient is irritable and irascible and wants to be left alone.

Nux vomica is also a good medicine for irritable people with headaches. The apparent cause of the headache is most often the best indication for *Nux,* since this medicine frequently suits the symptoms of headaches brought on by overeating, the use of alcohol, coffee or other drugs, or staying up too late and missing sleep. The person with a typical morning-hangover headache, who often has indulged in all of these pursuits, frequently is gratefully relieved with a dose or two of *Nux.* Such headaches are generally accompanied by an overall sick feeling and by digestive upsets. The sufferer may have a sour or bitter taste in the mouth in the morning, queasiness, nausea or vomiting (dry heaves and gas are especially typical *Nux* symptoms). The *Nux* headache may also be brought on by concentrated or prolonged mental work or by cold air or cold wind (many remedies cover headaches from cold, but *Nux* is an important one). In contrast to *Bryonia* headaches, those of *Nux* are worse in the morning, particularly upon first waking, and tend to get somewhat better after the person is up and about. As with most headaches, motion may aggravate the symptoms, but shaking the head is particularly painful (as in *Belladonna*). Lying on the painful side often makes the pain worse, and the sound of footsteps is particularly irritating to the *Nux*-headache patient. Wrapping the head up or being in a warm room may relieve the pain.

Pulsatilla headaches have also been associated with digestive upsets. They often come on after meals and particularly after eating warm, rich, or fatty foods or after eating ice cream. Nausea and vomiting frequently accompany a *Pulsatilla* headache. *Pulsatilla* is also a good medicine for headaches that occur in connection with menstrual periods (before, during, or especially when the period ends) or those that result from a frightening experience. The pain is most often felt in the forehead or on one side of the head and may change location frequently (as it does with *Sanguinaria*). Throbbing accompanies the headache. Although walking briskly may make the pain worse, generally there is relief with gentle motion, especially walking about slowly in the open air. Pressure relieves the pain and blowing the nose aggravates it. The *Pulsatilla* individual is emotionally mild and sensitive and may weep from the pains. Though a little irritable, the person is likely to want company and consolation.

Gelsemium headaches generally begin at the back of the head, often extending to the rest of the head or to the forehead. The person may feel as though a band or hood were bound tightly around the head. These symptoms are, of course, characteristic of muscle-contraction headaches. But *Gelsemium* is also one of the fairly few homeopathic medicines that clearly suit headaches preceded by dimness of vision or other visual disturbances, symptoms of migraines. Localized pain on the right side of the head is also covered by this remedy. The *Gelsemium* headache is not much affected by changes of temperature, but other environmental factors (light, noise, motion, jarring) aggravate it. Napping or, curiously, urinating relieves the pain. The person feels dull, tired, heavy, and apathetic. His eyes droop and he looks exhausted. He is not particularly irritable but wants to be left alone.

The headaches of *Iris* are also preceded or accompanied by dimness of vision or other changes in eyesight. The pain is felt in one side of the forehead, particularly the right side. Nausea and vomiting ensue, and the headache is worse after the vomiting. The pain is made better by walking in the open air. *Iris* has helped many people with periodic migraine headaches, such as those that return every weekend. Even if visual disturbance does not accompany the headache, *Iris* may help if its other symptoms fit.

Sanguinaria headaches typically begin in the back of the head but extend to and soon settle over the right eye or in the right side of the head. Right-sided headaches are covered by other medicines (*Iris* and *Gelsemium*, for instance) but *Sanguinaria* is especially noted for this symptom. The pain is sharp, splitting, knifelike, and sometimes throbbing. Once again, nausea and vomiting occur at the height of the pain, but unlike *Iris* headaches, those of *Sanguinaria* are relieved after vomiting. Motion aggravates the pain, whereas sleep and firm pressure relieve it. Like *Iris, Sanguinaria* suits headaches that recur in a consistent pattern, such as every seven days. Homeopathic reference texts do not mention *Sanguinaria* in connection with visual disturbances. However, if you have a classic, visual-aura migraine headache that also has the symptoms just mentioned, we certainly recommend that you use this medicine.

The headaches that need *Spigelia* are neurological and have stitching, burning, and pulsating pains, usually on frontal part of the head and often on the left side. Lying with the head propped

---

Beyond Home Care

Get Medical Care Immediately:

- for any very severe headache, particularly if it is unusual for you;
- for headache accompanied by stiff neck or high fever;
- for any headache that occurs after a head injury.

Get Medical Care Today:

- the first time you have a headache preceded or accompanied by visual disturbances, weakness of one side or part of the body, speech disorders, or dizziness. If you have had these symptoms previously, but their pattern has changed significantly, call or see your practitioner;
- for a headache lasting more than three or four days, even if mild (a call to your doctor may suffice);
- if a headache begins while you're taking medicine, including birth control pills.

See Your Practitioner Soon:

- for headaches that recur frequently, even if mild;
- for headaches that are consistently worse in the morning or upon waking.

up makes the pains better; stooping, motion, noise, and cold stormy weather make them worse. Washing with cold water can feel good, but the pain is usually worse after you finish. In general, the head pains are made worse by warmth and temporarily better by cold (for other pain symptoms of *Spigelia* the reverse is true). A stiff neck and shoulders accompany the headache and make motion very painful. The person may also experience severe pain in and around the eyes and extending deep into the sockets.

CHAPTER 12
Allergies

Allergic symptoms occur when the body's immune system overreacts to substances in the environment. When the body is healthy, the immune system's ability to identify and remove foreign substances enables it to fight off infecting germs, neutralize poisons, and destroy cancer cells. During an allergic reaction, however, these normally protective defenses are triggered by innocuous substances such as foods, pollens, animal hairs, medicines, and so forth, and uncomfortable, sometimes dangerous symptoms are produced. The most common symptoms of allergic reactions include skin eruptions, stuffy or runny nose, and wheezing or coughing. We cover common allergic skin conditions (contactc dermatitis, hives, and eczema) and respiratory disorders (upper respiratory allergies and asthma) in this chapter. Severe, generalized allergic reactions, called *anaphylaxis,* are rare (see the section on shock in chapter 14).

In a strict medical sense, allergies are reactions to specific foreign substances. However, the immune system can also produce similar symptoms when triggered by nonspecific factors such as temperature or weather changes, overexertion, stress, strong emotions, or infectious illness; sometimes the symptoms seem to develop "by themselves."

In either case, homeopathy offers a uniquely effective way to treat the person with allergies and related conditions. From the homeopathic perspective, the basic problem is an imbalance in the system as a whole, which leads to the oversensitive state. It is sensible to avoid substances or other influences that trigger symptoms. Often, however, identifying exactly what causes the reaction is nearly impossible. Many times, too, it turns out to be something you just can't avoid completely. Moreover, the underlying weakness remains; the symptoms return as soon as the substance is encountered again.

Professional constitutional homeopathic treatment can help the system correct its imbalance and help free it from its sensitivity. In the home, homeopathic medicines may be used when acute, short-lived allergy symptoms occur in people who are otherwise healthy. Even when constitutional care is needed for recurrent allergies, home treatment during a particularly bad outbreak of symptoms may offer great relief. If you are receiving constitutional care, please consult with your homeopath before using home treatment.

Contact Dermatitis

Any itching skin eruption triggered by exposure to allergenic substances is called *contact dermatitis*. The most familiar kind is the rash that appears after contact with or exposure to poison oak, ivy, or sumach. Other common causes of contact dermatitis include other plants, cosmetics, jewelry, and rubber. Some diaper rashes are triggered by contact allergic reactions to the laundry detergent or to chemicals in disposable diapers, and others occur as a reaction to contact with irritating urine. Contact rashes may become infected with bacteria or fungi; otherwise the main concern is the itching and unattractive appearance.

Diagnosis of contact dermatitis depends on careful attention to the details of how the rash appeared. Think about what may have touched the skin at the site of the rash, and try to recall any new household chemicals, toiletries, or clothing in use. PABA, found in sunscreen lotions, and benzocaine, found in many topical pain relievers and antiseptics, are frequent offenders.

General Home Care

Once you know the rash's cause, avoiding it for a week or two should clear it up. There are many topical treatments advised for poison-oak rashes and the like, but none have been consistently successful in our experience. Some of the most promising include liberal applications of the juice of the plantain (*Plantago*) or *Grindelia* plants (either fresh or as tinctures available from homeopathic pharmacies) or green clay powder (available in health food stores). Calamine lotion and the like feel cooling but don't really relieve much itching. Hydrocortisone creams are now offered over-the-counter as poison-oak remedies, but even these potent drugs rarely help.

Homeopathic Medicines

Homeopathic medicines can work to help the body relieve itching and speed healing of the rash. Some of our severely poison-oak-sensitive patients have told us that the homeopathic treatment brought faster and more complete improvement than powerful oral doses of steroid hormones.

Choose a medicine and give it two to three times a day for up to three days. Stop as soon as there is significant improvement in the itching or the rash.

Homeopathic medicines made from *Rhus toxicodendron* (poison ivy) or *Rhus diversiloba* (poison oak) can be very effective for people who are reacting to these plants, or who have contact dermatitis caused by other substances. If no other medicine is clearly indicated, you can try one of these. The *Rhus* patient has burning, itching eruptions, and the discomfort is aggravated by scratching, open air, night, and the warmth of the bed. He gets relief from the itching by immersing the area in near-scalding water. There are fluid-filled blisters with great inflammation. The patient is generally restless, irritable, and anxious.

With *Croton tig.* eruptions, there is a great deal of blistering and inflammation but less burning than with the *Rhus* rash. If the eruption is mild, gentle scratching or rubbing relieves the itching, but as it gets worse, it is painful and tender and the patient can't stand to touch it. The *Croton tig.* rash tends to be worst on the scalp, around the eyes, and on the genitals.

Anacardium should also be considered when there are large blisters filled with yellow fluid. The face may be prominently affected by the eruption.

Bryonia can be helpful when the rash is mainly made up of fine, dry bumps, especially on the face. The symptoms are made worse by moving around, and the person is irritable and wants to be left alone.

Sepia is also a possibility when the rash is dry (there may be tiny blisters but not large ones). A warm room may help relieve itching, but getting warm in bed makes it worse. The rash may have a brownish or reddish color, and scaling may be evident.

Graphites should be thought of when there is much oozing of sticky, honey-colored fluid from the eruptions. Itching is worse at night and in warmth.

Sulphur may help no matter what the rash looks like, if the general characteristics of the medicine are marked. Itching is worse in warmth and at night, and usually the person is sensitive to heat and feels warm.

Once the rash has begun to subside and itching is less intense, apply one part *Calendula* tincture diluted with three parts water with a cotton swab several times a day. The skin will heal much faster, particularly if it has been open and raw from blistering.

Beyond Home Care

Consult the section on impetigo in chapter 13 if signs of infection (pus, swelling, spreading redness) appear.

Hives

Hives are red, raised swellings, or welts, that appear suddenly with intense itching. The individual welts are generally a half-inch across or larger, and they may run together to form large patches of raised, puffy skin.

Hives may be triggered by food, food additives, medicines, insect venoms, anything cold touching the skin, rubbing or scratching the skin, and emotions. Often the precipitating cause is never found. The eruption lasts from several hours to a day or so and disappears as quickly as it came, leaving no trace. Most people get hives only once or twice in a lifetime, but some get them recurrently.

Hives are only a nuisance unless the swelling involves the respiratory passages. Occasionally, severe allergic reactions cause hivelike swellings in the throat that impede breathing.

General Home Care

Since attacks of hives are generally self-limited, little treatment is really necessary. Applying a cool sponge to the affected area, may relieve itching and help bring down the swelling, unless the hives are caused by cold.

Homeopathic Medicines

Recurrent outbreaks are a constitutional problem and should be treated by a homeopath. During an isolated case of hives choose from among the following remedies.

The medicine most likely to help the person with hives is *Apis*. The hives are intensely itchy and usually aggravated by warmth. They are worse at night and come on during perspiration, after exercise, or when the body becomes hot; they may begin after any change in weather. *Apis* is particularly indicated when the hives cause swelling around the eyes.

If neither of the medicines listed below is strongly indicated, use *Apis* whether or not its characteristic symptoms are present. Give a dose of the 30th potency every three hours, stopping as soon as improvement begins. Often a single dose is enough to bring rapid improvement.

Urtica urens, the stinging nettle, should also be considered. As with *Apis,* the hives are made worse by warmth or exercise, in this case especially if the exercise is particularly strenuous. Bathing may bring on the eruption, and the patient may get relief by lying down.

Beyond Home Care

Get Medical Care Immediately:

- if the hives involve the throat, or if a sense of constriction in the throat is felt, even mildly. Swelling may suddenly increase and interfere with breathing.

Give *Rhus tox.* if rubbing or scratching, cold weather, or getting wet seems to bring on the welts. Welts may also form during perspiration.

Atopic Dermatitis (Eczema)

The term *eczema* describes any rash that reddens and inflames the skin, causing bumps and tiny blisters, oozing, crusting, or dryness and thickening of the skin. Although many skin conditions cause eczematous eruptions, eczema is most often thought of as synonymous with *atopic dermatitis,* a chronic skin disorder related to allergies. Because it is a chronic, deeply rooted condition, atopic dermatitis should be treated constitutionally by a skilled homeopathic practitioner.

Conventional treatment with corticosteroid-hormone creams should be avoided if at all possible. These medications are absorbed into the circulation, and when applied to large areas of raw skin, they can profoundly affect the body's hormonal balance. Homeopaths are also concerned about the way they so strongly suppress symptoms, since the body may need to react to the imbalance with deeper, more serious symptoms.

General Home Care

Don't bathe too often, and use as little soap as possible. Irritating fabrics like wool should be avoided. Launder clothes in mild detergents or plain water. Be sure to keep the skin well lubricated with bland, unmedicated cream or lotion.

Upper Respiratory Tract Allergies

Many people suffer from allergic reactions that involve the nose, throat, eyes, and ears. The symptoms of these allergies include sneezing, runny or stuffy nose, itchy and watery eyes, as well as itching of the throat, roof of the mouth, or ears, or any combination of these. Pollens, dust, animal fur, and other inhaled allergens are most often associated with respiratory allergies, though foods and other substances may also be involved. Seasonal reaction to high levels of pollen in the air, which prevails when weeds and trees are in bloom, is called *hay fever.*

Standard treatment of upper-respiratory allergies includes antihistamines, decongestants, and desensitization shots. Both antihistamines and decongestants directly suppress the body's defenses. Not only do the symptoms come right back as soon as the drugs wear off, but such suppression may force the system to create deeper symptoms to handle the underlying imbalance. Antihistamines cause drowsiness and often dryness of the mouth. When decongestants wear off there is a "rebound" effect, and the symptoms become worse than before. Avoid these medicines if possible.

Desensitization therapy (allergy shots) involves frequent injections of known allergens in minute amounts. The dose is gradually increased until the person can tolerate exposure to the allergens in daily life. Though this approach makes more sense to us than symptom suppression, it has its problems. The shots occasionally cause severe allergic reactions requiring emergency treatment. Exposure to allergens by injection does not occur naturally. And the treatment only works for the allergens used in the injections; the underlying tendency toward allergic reactions is not addressed. We recommend you try homeopathic treatment first.

General Home Care

Avoiding pollens, animal hairs, and other things that stimulate your allergies is of course important when possible. Rinsing mucus membranes of the nose and eyes with normal saline solution (it should be sterile if used in the eyes) to remove pollen granules and other allergens may bring substantial relief. You should drink ample amounts of water. Inhaling water vapor from a humidifier can help open swollen air passages.

Homeopathic Medicines

Constitutional homeopathic treatment is indicated if symptoms of upper-respiratory allergies are recurrent. Still, you can use homeopathic medicines at home to get through the worst part of an allergy attack. Consult your homeopath first if you are being treated constitutionally.

Read the descriptions of medicines in the chapter on colds, especially those of *Nux vomica, Arsenicum, Allium cepa,* and *Euphrasia,* as well as those that follow here. Give one dose of the most appropriate medicine and observe the reaction. If symptoms improve, give no more medicine until they return. If there is no reaction after four hours, repeat the medicine and allow four more hours before trying a new medicine.

Once you find a medicine that helps, you can use it to treat severe symptoms up to three times a day but for no more than a week. Be sure not to give any medicine whenever there is still improvement from the previous dose.

Sabadilla covers the typical symptoms of hay-fever allergies, including copious, watery nasal discharge, spasmodic sneezing, itching in the nose, and red, runny eyes. All these symptoms are improved by being outdoors or walking in the open air. There may be a sensation like a lump in the throat along with a constant urge to swallow.

Wyethia is indicated when upper-respiratory allergies are accompanied by intense, urgent itching of the back part of the roof of the mouth or itching behind the nose. The nose, nasal passages, and throat feel dry in spite of a continuous, burning, watery flow from the nose.

Arsenicum, Euphrasia, Nux vomica, or *Sabadilla* may be indicated if the symptoms progress to include mild wheezing.

Asthma

Asthma occurs when the breathing passages in the chest narrow from contraction of the passages' muscular walls, swelling of their linings, and accumulation of thick mucus within the tubes. The narrowed breathing tubes impede the normal flow of air into and, especially, out of the lungs. The chest feels tight and the person is short of breath, wheezes, and must breathe rapidly with much greater effort.

The worst symptoms of an asthma attack may run their course within a day or two, usually clearing without treatment. But you

Conventional medical treatment of asthma includes avoidance of known allergens or other triggering substances, desensitization shots (see section on upper-respiratory tract allergies) if specific allergens have been identified, and various drugs. A fairly severe, acute attack of asthma is usually treated with an injection of *epinephrine* (adrenaline), which forces the tightened breathing tubes to relax, or with another bronchodilating drug. For maintenance of recurrent asthma, drugs containing theophylline or epinephrine-related chemicals are generally used. These also make the breathing passages open and relax, and they may be given orally. Frequent side effects include irritability, restlessness, insomnia, and palpitations, though these can be minimized if the dose is carefully adjusted. Even stronger drugs such as steroid hormones are given if others fail to control asthma.

Though all conventional drugs carry the risk of side effects, sometimes they are simply necessary. Details of treatment must be worked out with your practitioner, but we recommend appropriate conventional medications be used if an asthma attack remains severe for more than a brief period or whenever there is doubt that the person is getting enough oxygen.

General Home Care

During an attack of wheezing, drinking plenty of liquids is extremely important to replacing water lost through rapid breathing and increased perspiration (see the section on dehydration in the chapter 8 on digestive problems for more information). The liquids also help loosen sticky mucus in the breathing passages. Relaxation practices often help. Breathing exercises (your practitioner can demonstrate them) are valuable both during acute attacks and when the patient gets asthma recurrently.

Homeopathic Medicines

Asthma is often a deep-seated, genetically determined illness, but most asthmatics have gone through periods when symptoms were absent or minimal, even though no obvious environmental changes had occurred. Constitutional homeopathic treatment can make these periods of freedom from asthma more frequent and longer lasting. Though occasional setbacks for which standard drugs must be used can be expected, overall improvement will come.

Once the diagnosis of asthma is established, and once you are familiar with the pattern of symptoms, you can use homeopathy at home for mild-to-moderate, acute asthma symptoms. If you are receiving constitutional care, consult your homeopath first.

Give the first three doses of the medicine you select every hour or two, but stop as soon as there is real improvement. If there is no improvement an hour after the third dose, try a second medicine, using the same method. If it is helping, you may repeat it whenever symptoms worsen, but not more often than once every two hours or ten times in two days. Until the symptoms disappear completely, you should be in contact with your health practitioner at least once a day.

The strongest indications for the use of *Arsenicum* are fearfulness, restlessness, weakness, and aggravation of the symptoms at or after midnight. It's not at all surprising that the asthmatic grows frightened when he can't get his breath, and *Arsenicum* suits the restless agitation typical of this state. The patient tosses and turns or suddenly springs out of bed to relieve the anxiety and to catch a deep breath. In spite of the urge to move about, a profound weakness often develops, and the person may become too weak to continue his restless behavior and may be unable to move much at all. Most *Arsenicum* patients have the worst time with wheezing and shortness of breath between midnight and 3 A.M. If other symptoms suggest the medicine, however, don't hesitate to try it just because the asthma is worse at some other time of day or night. There may be accompanying cough or cold or hay-fever symptoms. Most *Arsenicum* patients feel quite chilly and are relieved by warmth generally. They tend to be quite thirsty, sometimes for frequent sips of water.

If the asthmatic is sweet and affectionate or perhaps tearful and clingy, feels oppressed by warm and stuffy rooms, and has little thirst, *Pulsatilla* is the probable remedy, no matter what the respiratory symptoms are. On the other hand, you may give *Pulsatilla* when it is indicated by specific asthma symptoms, including wheezing that begins or is worse in the evening or at night. There is usually an accumulation of phlegm in the chest that must be coughed out (see the description in chapter 4 on colds and coughs). The asthma may be worse after eating, especially eating fatty or rich foods.

Ipecac is similarly suited to those whose asthma is accompanied by a great deal of phlegm in the chest. The respiratory distress may be spasmodic and severe, with marked wheezing. But you may hear, in addition to the wheezing, much rattling of mucus in the chest as the person breathes. Coughing is common and sounds rattly from mucus deep in the chest. The cough may come in intense spasms that continue until there is vomiting of food or mucus. The asthma may be worse at night. The patient is often nauseated, and vomiting is common even when there is no coughing (see chapter 8 on digestive problems). Exhausted by the illness, the person looks pale and quite sick. Many of these symptoms are similar to those of *Pulsatilla,* but with *Ipecac,* the buildup of mucus is even greater and the characteristic mental symptoms of *Pulsatilla* are not prominent.

Beyond Home Care

Get Medical Care Immediately:

- for any severe shortness of breath;
- if shortness of breath is accompanied by severe sore throat with difficulty swallowing, or if you notice that a wheezing child is drooling a great deal.

Get Medical Care Today:

- for a first occurrence of wheezing, or if the pattern of wheezing is different from the established one;
- whenever wheezing occurs in children under two years old. For anyone over this age, you should consult with your practitioner ahead of time so you know how to handle recurrences of asthma that do follow the person's established pattern.

Spongia, on the other hand, suits those whose asthma is dry with little or no phlegm in the chest. Breathing is labored and noisy, sounding like whistling or sawing (typical of asthma but most pronounced when *Spongia* is the remedy). Often the asthma begins after the person has been chilled or was coming down with a cold. There may be sudden onset of wheezing with a feeling of suffocation just as the person begins to fall asleep, or the wheezing may be worse after sleep. Shortness of breath is made worse by lying down and by every motion, and it gets better when the person leans the head back. Warm food or drinks may help relieve the wheezing. A dry barking or croupy cough may accompany the wheezing.

Bryonia may be called for if the symptoms are typical of the remedy in general: aggravation caused by motion is pronounced, and the patient is warm, thirsty, and probably irritable. The wheezing is dry in character with little phlegm.

Chamomilla should be considered for people with asthma, especially children, when they strongly display the irritability typical of the medicine. You should also consider *Chamomilla* if the asthma began after anger.

CHAPTER 13

Skin Problems and
Related Disorders

The skin is the largest organ of the body. It covers an area of some 3,000 square inches on an average adult, and one third of all the circulating blood is supplied to the skin. Many important physiological functions are performed by the skin. It helps to regulate body temperature and participates in the control of fluid balance. Nerve endings sensitive to temperature, pain, touch, and pressure are located in the skin. The outer layer of the skin produces an acidic *mantle,* or covering, that inhibits the growth of disease-causing bacteria. The skin is also an organ of elimination of fluids, minerals, and various biochemicals.

Homeopaths believe the skin has other functions as well. According to our understanding, the body uses the skin to "eliminate" internal imbalance by expressing it in the appearance of skin symptoms. Homeopaths consider the appearance of a skin disorder an indication that the body is moving the level of physiological imbalance to the surface.

Since the skin is the most external organ of the body, skin troubles are seen as the healthiest symptoms the body can produce as it heals from the inside out. They show that the body is keeping the imbalance as far away from the vital organs as possible.

Therefore, we encourage you not to look at skin symptoms as nuisances that should be done away with. There may well be a reason for their appearance, and they may represent a body's healthy response to stress. Certainly you should correct any conditions affecting hygiene, diet, or psychological stress that contribute to your susceptibility, but try to avoid medicines that suppress symptoms. Seek homeopathic treatment that helps rouse the body's defenses to fully restore balance.

Many people with common skin problems can be treated with simple home-care measures and homeopathic medicines. In this chapter we cover boils, styes, impetigo, herpes, shingles, ringworm, yeast infections, and warts (hives and contact dermatitis, such as poison oak, are covered in chapter 12 on allergies). We only have space enough for outline descriptions of these conditions. If you're not positive what the problem is, you'll have to rely on other medical self-care books or a visit to your medical professional. People who have chronic skin troubles—such as psoriasis, eczema (see the chapter on allergies), or frequently recurring infections—should be treated constitutionally by a professional homeopath.

Boils, Abscesses, and Other Skin Infections

Boils and other skin infections occur when the skin's first levels of defense are breached. The outer layer of the skin serves as a barrier that is usually impenetrable to germs. Once disease-causing bacteria have passed through this outer barrier, they are quickly recognized by the immune defenses and attacked. More blood is brought to the area to increase these immune responses. At the same time, changes in the skin tissue occur that serve to wall off the infected area from nearby healthy skin, preventing the spread of the bacteria.

Boils are one way the interactions of germs and the body's defenses become visibly manifest. As the infection/inflammation process progresses, the skin becomes red, swollen, and warm because of the increased blood brought to the area. Stretching of the swollen skin may cause much pain. The inflammation may resolve without further complication, but when it does not eliminate and absorb the infection quickly, the walling-off process continues, and pus forms in a central cavity of the developing boil. Pus is a mixture of fluid from the blood, dead white blood cells, and bacteria. As the inflammatory process continues to battle aggressive germs, boils can become as large as an inch or two in diameter; a carbuncle is a particularly large boil with multiple centers of pus formation.

In time, the boil comes to a head at the surface of the skin, eventually opening to allow the pus to escape. Once the boil has ruptured and released the pus, pain is relieved immediately and the infection heals rapidly. But sometimes the infected material is permanently enclosed in a protective capsule, from which it may be absorbed by the body. The healthy function of these defenses results in complete healing of the skin or, at worst, a small lump where the infected tissue has been enclosed and reabsorbed.

Any localized collection of pus encapsulated in a cavity is called an *abscess*. Boils are abscesses in the skin, but abscesses themselves can occur in many other parts of the body. Other abscesses that you can often treat at home include infections around the finger and toenails (whitlows), and styes (these are covered later in this chapter).

Boils are usually not serious health problems if the infection remains confined to the immediate area of the swelling. But if the body's defenses cannot contain the bacteria within the boil, the germs invade the surrounding tissues, where they can spread more quickly and sometimes enter the bloodstream to cause generalized illness.

Cellulitis is the term for an infection spreading within the skin and underlying tissues that is not walled within a specific area. The first hint of cellulitis is often the presence of red streaks extending away from a boil, an abscess, or any other skin infection like impetigo (see the following section). The body continues to fight the infection with inflammation and immunity defenses but, until these defenses prevail, cellulitis develops as a puffy, red swelling that extends from the original infection and that feels warm to the touch. The inflammation of cellulitis is usually too diffuse to cause pus to form anywhere but in the original boil.

When bacteria enter the bloodstream in significant numbers, a generalized illness may ensue. The person feels sick with fever, muscle aches, and severe headaches. Shock may occur.

General Home Care

The best home treatment for simple boils is to aid the body's inflammatory defenses with hot compresses or soakings. Applying heat to a well-localized skin infection brings the area even more blood to help kill germs, to remove dead cells and debris, and to begin the healing process. The heat helps bring the boil to a head and hastens the discharge of pus. Keeping a nutritious diet and getting plenty of rest are also essential.

Homeopathic Medicines

Homeopathic medicines help increase the body's natural protective responses to the infection. If the proper medicine is given early enough, the infection will resolve before pus ever forms. Given later, the medicines will help ripen the infection so that the pus is eliminated early and completely.

When treating a person with a boil, carbuncle, felon, or abscess of any kind, give the one, best-indicated medicine from the following list every three to four hours while redness, swelling, and pain are most acute. Give at least three doses before changing medicines if there seems to be no effect. Once improvement begins, continue giving the medicine three times a day until pus is no longer being discharged, swelling has clearly improved, and redness is diminishing.

Use *Belladonna* during the early stages of any localized boil or abscess. There is painful, bright red, hot swelling but little or no pus formation yet. Throbbing in the developing boil is characteristic. Given early, *Belladonna* frequently helps the body arrest the development of the boil so that healing occurs before pus ever forms.

If *Belladonna* does not help, or if treatment has begun more than twenty-four hours after the onset of symptoms, choose from one of the following medicines:

Before pus has clearly formed, *Hepar sulph.* often helps the body heal the inflammation by absorbing the boil altogether. If the young boil is very painful and tender to the touch, *Hepar* is especially well indicated. *Hepar* is also useful after pus has formed, again, if the inflamed part is very painful. *Hepar* boils are typically tender to the slightest touch and extremely sensitive to cold air or cold applications. There may be throbbing or, more often, sharp or sticking pains, as if a splinter were stuck in the painful part. *Hepar* and *Silica* are both good medicines for boils that are slow to heal, even after pus has drained; choose between the two on the basis of the symptoms.

Once pus has definitely formed and gathered, *Mercurius* is the

---

Beyond Home Care

Antibiotics are of little use in the treatment of simple boils, since they do not penetrate very well the central cavity of the boil, where the infection is most active. When a boil or abscess is located on the face or head, there is some chance the infection will spread to the brain, and in such cases antibiotics are indeed recommended. Antibiotics may be a good idea if a fever accompanies the boil. In conventional medical practice, cellulitis is treated with antibiotics because of the risk it may continue spreading to other areas of the body or to the blood; this is also appropriate.

Once a boil has come to a head and pus has clearly formed, the healing process may sometimes be hastened by surgically opening the skin to allow the pus to drain. This procedure must be performed by your health practitioner.

Get Medical Care Immediately:

- if there is high fever, severe headache, or stiffness of the neck.

See Your Practitioner Today:

- if the infection is accompanied by fever, malaise, or muscle aches;
- if a boil is located on the head or face;
- if redness or swelling is spreading from the boil area;
- if pain is severe or the boil is extremely swollen with pus;
- if the boil is not improving with home treatment after forty-eight to seventy-two hours;
- if the boil has opened but does not appear to be healing after a week.

likely remedy. This medicine helps bring the abscess to a head and speeds the drainage of pus. The boil is painful but no so sensitive to touch as the *Hepar* one. Warmth may aggravate the pain.

Silica is suitable for those boils or abscesses that are slow to heal, even though pus is freely draining. Compared with the *Hepar* boil, that of *Silica* is less sensitive and painful, though there may be relief with warmth. Similarly, give *Silica* two or three times a day after a boil or whitlow has been lanced and drained. *Silica* is also indicated when a boil comes on slowly or redness and swelling persist for several days without the development of pus. Firm, red cystic lumps that persist after a boil has mostly healed often disappear after a dose or two of *Silica* 30c or if *Silica* 6x is taken once or twice daily for a week or so.

Arsenicum is indicated at any stage of an abscess if there is great burning pain clearly relieved by warm applications. The general symptoms of *Arsenicum* may be present.

Choose *Lachesis* if the abscess and surrounding skin become bluish or purplish. Typically, pus is dark and thin, and the abscess is tender to touch. Be especially careful to discontinue this medicine as soon as improvement has begun.

Styes

A *stye* is an infected pimple or small boil on the eyelid. The germs, usually *Staphylococci,* grow in the oil or sweat glands of the eyelid. The inflammation surfaces at the margin of the lid as a tender, red swelling. Within a few days the stye comes to a head and then opens to let pus drain. Pimples similar to styes may also form on the inside of the eyelid and are basically the same type of infection. Occasionally, however, these infections on the inner eyelid may spread and involve the whole lid.

Although they can be quite painful, styes are rarely dangerous and they usually heal by themselves. Occasionally a stye does not heal completely and leaves behind a firm, red cystic lump in the eyelid. These cysts are not painful themselves, but in some cases they rub against the eye and new acute styes may develop within them recurrently. Constitutional homeopathic treatment can help strengthen the body and eliminate susceptibility to recurrent styes.

General Home Care

Soak a clean washcloth in warm water and apply it to the affected eye for ten to fifteen minutes three or four times a day. The warmer the water, the better—though you should make sure it isn't hot enough to burn the skin. Expect the stye to improve within forty-eight hours.

Homeopathic Medicines

Styes are small abscesses distinguished by their location in the eyelids. Any of the medicines listed in the section on boils and abscesses may be helpful, if the other symptoms so indicate.

Give a dose of the best-indicated medicine every six to eight hours for up to three days, but stop as soon as you notice improvement. Repeat the dose only if the symptoms get worse again or if there has been no further improvement for twenty-four hours.

Pulsatilla is one of the most commonly used medicines for people with styes, and it should be given if no other medicine is clearly indicated. Most often, the stye occurs on the upper lids. The stye may not be particularly painful, in spite of the inflammation. It comes to a head and discharges a yellow-to-green pus.

Beyond Home Care

Get Medical Care Today:

- if vision is affected in any way;
- if the stye is accompanied by fever, headache, loss of appetite, or lethargy;
- if the swelling is located on or directed toward the inside of the eyelid;
- if the stye persists for more than forty-eight hours despite the use of warm applications and homeopathic treatment.

Note: Consult the section on conjunctivitis if the white of the eye becomes inflamed.

Hepar sulph. is effective when the stye is hypersensitive to touch, cold air, and cold applications. The pain is throbbing in character, or it may feel as if a splinter were in the eyelid. The pain is relieved by warm applications.

Apis also covers painful styes, especially those that burn and sting and are made worse by heat or warm applications. *Apis* should also be thought of if the entire lid becomes red and swollen.

Graphites styes are painful but not so tender to touch as those of *Hepar.* Thick yellow material may be discharged from the stye. Crusts, scales, and sores on the eyelids are typical of *Graphites.*

Staphysagria is indicated when styes come out in crops, one after another, over a period of weeks. The problem may begin after the person suffers nervous exhaustion.

Consider *Lycopodium* if the stye is near the inner corner of the eye.

Firm cysts that remain in the eyelid after the acute stage of a style often heal following a dose or two of the 30th potency of *Staphysagria* or *Silica.*

Impetigo

Impetigo is a highly contagious, superficial bacterial infection of the skin caused by *Streptococcus* and *Staphylococcus* bacteria. The eruption consists of small, red, raised bumps that quickly develop into tiny blisters, which then pop and ooze a sticky fluid and leave raw, red sores. Soon the sores are covered with a sticky, golden yellow crust. The infection can spread rapidly, as the bacteria are carried on fingers, clothing, and so on. Crops of crusty sores may quickly develop. Children are more prone to impetigo than are adults, and they can easily pass the contagious germs on to their playmates.

Impetigo is most commonly located on the face. Sores frequently appear on the cheeks, about the lips, and at the nostrils. The sores' appearance is similar to that of cold sores or herpes, but impetigo spreads more rapidly, does not confine itself to one area of the body, and does not affect the inner lips or inside the mouth. Any doubt about which infection is responsible for a given eruption can be cleared up by taking a culture.

Impetigo sores rarely hurt, and eventually most people overcome the infection on their own. But in the meantime the sores may become widespread, and other people may become infected. There are also a number of complications that can develop. These include infection of the deeper layers of skin (see the discussion of cellulitis in the section on boils); and a kidney disease that is caused by the immune system's reaction to *Streptococcus* germs. Only certain strains of the strep bacteria trigger this disease (called *glomerulonephritis*), so several members of a family, neighborhood, or school group may all come down with it after catching impetigo. Symptoms include malaise, loss of appetite, nausea, headache, reduced urine production, and puffiness and swelling of the face and extremities. This illness almost always clears up without permanent problems.

General Home Care

Preventing impetigo is difficult, but you should try to keep your children from playing with others who have the infection. If you or a family member has impetigo, avoid touching the sores, and wash your hands immediately if you do. Use warm soakings to remove the crusts, and then wash them and the surrounding skin with gentle soap and water. *Calendula* tincture (diluted 3:1 with sterile water or normal saline) should then be painted on the sores with a sterile cotton swab. Allow the sores to dry, and leave them exposed to the air. Topical antibiotics such as Neosporin rarely help, and creams may delay healing.

Homeopathic Medicines

Impetigo should respond quickly to homeopathic treatment; you should notice improvement in both general and skin symptoms within twelve to twenty-four hours after you first give the medicine. Give the remedy every four to six hours, but stop as soon as any improvement begins. Switch medicines if there is no change after a full day, but be sure to check the "Beyond Home Care" recommendations regularly.

Antimonium crudum covers the classic symptoms of impetigo. There is an oozing eruption with the formation of thick yellow crusts. The eruption is worse on the face. The individual sores begin to run together into larger patches. They may seem to spread or look more inflamed after bathing. In general the *Antimomium crudum* patient is irritable and may not be able to stand being looked at. The tongue may have a thick white coat.

The person who has impetigo with markedly scabby, oozy eruptions needs *Graphites*. This is especially true if the liquid in the sores is sticky and has the color, though not necessarily the thickness, of honey. The sores are most likely to be worse around the mouth or nose.

Rhus tox. may be indicated when impetigo is maddeningly itchy. The blisters are small but appear in clusters. There may be itching as well as stinging or tingling in the sores. The discomfort is better when the patient is moving around. The discharge from the crusty, oozing sores is sometimes dark but translucent.

Mercurius is indicated if the sores are open and especially deep. The typical yellowish crusts may form, especially around the mouth or on the scalp, but the discharge is of pus rather than of translucent

---

Beyond Home Care

Conventional practitioners use oral antibiotics, including erythromycin and synthetic penicillin drugs such as dicloxacillin. Antibiotics do not prevent glomerulonephritis, but they do kill the germs and help prevent spread of the infection. Therefore they are a good public health measure, if those from whom you caught the impetigo had glomerulonephritis.

Get Medical Care Today:

- if there are more than three or four sores or if the sores are large or painful;
- if there is fever, malaise, or muscle aches;
- if redness or swelling extends from the sores;
- if you are infected after exposure to others who have had glomerulonephritis;
- if the sores do not improve within forty-eight to seventy-two hours.

liquid and is likely to smell bad. The discharge may also be streaked with a little blood. Swelling of the lymph nodes of the face and neck is common.

Hepar can be a good medicine for the person with impetigo if the sores are especially sore to the touch and sensitive to cold. The scabs are often soft and break apart easily. As with *Mercurius*, there may well be pus formation and swelling of the glands. Also similar to *Mercurius*, the sores may be deep and may bleed a little. The typical *Hepar* patient is extremely irritable.

If the sores burn or feel painfully raw and feel better in warmth or with warm applications, *Arsenicum* is probably indicated. The sores tend to look dark. They exude a thin watery fluid or sometimes pus.

Herpes Simplex

Herpes is an infection of the skin and nerves caused by a small virus related to the chicken pox virus. After exposure to the germ, usually in three to six days, the characteristic eruption breaks out, appearing as groups of tiny blisters (vesicles) surrounded by red, angry, inflamed skin. Each individual vesicle is only a millimeter long, while the patches of grouped vesicles are usually half an inch in diameter or less.

At first, each tiny vesicle is filled with a clear liquid, but this may become white or yellow pus. After a day or so the vesicles pop and merge, leaving a shallow, raw, red sore, which in turn scabs, eventually dries up, and heals.

There are two strains of the herpes virus: Type I usually infects the face and mouth (cold sores or fever blisters), while Type II is most often responsible for eruptions on the genitals and surrounding areas. The virus enters through the skin or mucous membranes. It can only survive within the human body, so infection is passed from one person to the next through direct contact with the sores or by being carried briefly on something warm and moist such as fingers or a towel. Recently it has been shown that the virus can survive in bath water or hot tubs, but it is quickly destroyed when dried. Herpes is most contagious when the vesicles are present or just after they have popped, but it should be considered infectious until the sores are completely healed.

Once you contract herpes, the virus lives permanently in the infected nerve cells. It is estimated that 95% of the population harbors the Type I germ. Herpes eruptions are often recurrent; they may break out at regular intervals or in response to a particular stimulus, such as sunlight or sexual activity. The first time the sores appear is usually the worst, as they form in larger, more numerous, and more painful groups of vesicles. About a third of the people with first-time herpes experience fever, muscle aches, headache, and other general symptoms suggestive of a viral illness. These symptoms rarely return with later outbreaks, but generally the sores themselves hurt or itch somewhat.

Herpes is not a serious disease in healthy adults, though it can be painful and annoying. Most people adjust to the virus fairly well, and recurrences generally become less frequent over time. Homeopaths consider most cases of herpes as representing relatively mild illness, the same as the majority of skin diseases. The body's defense mechanism is able to keep the level of physiological imbalance, as manifested in the susceptibility to the herpes infection, at the very periphery of the body, an achievement consistent with good health.

In contrast to the ordinary form of this illness, herpes can be a serious, generalized infection if it occurs in newborn babies or people whose immunity is too weak. Preventing herpes is critical, and mothers prone to recurrent herpes outbreaks should be observed closely by their practitioner. No one with an active herpes sore of either type should be allowed to handle a baby unless the sores are completely covered by clean clothing or a fresh bandage, and then only if the person bathes and washes his hands thoroughly before touching the child. People who suffer from debilitating illnesses or who have seriously decreased resistance are also susceptible to severe herpes infection, and the same precautions apply.

More common is herpes infection of the eye. The symptoms, including redness and watering, are similar to those of ordinary viral conjunctivitis (see the chapter on colds), but there is, in addition, marked pain and reduced vision. Herpes sores may or may not be present on the face. This is a serious condition that can cause permanent damage to eyesight if untreated. It represents an emergency and must be treated by a medical professional immediately (see "Beyond Home Care" in the chapter 4 section on conjunctivitis).

In conventional medicine, new antiviral drugs, such as acyclovir, are now being used against herpes. These medicines more effectively treat the rash than previous nonspecific measures. Still, the homeopath's concern is that drug treatment only suppresses the eruption and thereby blocks the body's best strategy for dealing with the underlying imbalance.

General Home Care

Keep the eruption and surrounding skin clean and dry, and cover it with a dry gauze bandage to protect it from injury and bacteria when you go out. Examine the rash to be sure that a bacterial infection isn't taking hold (indicated by a great deal of pus or redness spreading from around the sores). Take special care to eat well and get ample rest.

Homeopathic Medicines

Apply *Calendula tincture,* diluted 3:1 with water, several times a day after the sores have opened; this helps the skin heal a little more quickly.

Use oral homeopathic medicines to treat a person with herpes only during an acute outbreak. Give a dose of the medicine that best fits the symptoms twice a day for two or three days, stopping if any noticeable improvement occurs. Change to a new medicine after two days if the person is not better.

Rhus tox. is an important remedy for people with herpes. Small inflamed blisters appearing in clusters and filled with a yellowish, watery fluid are typical of herpes and of this medicine, as are intense burning and itching. Outbreaks may be accompanied by a general feeling of sickness and achiness, with aches and pains improved by moving around. *Rhus tox., along with Ars., Nat. mur.,* and *Hepar,* is a primary medicine for people with cold sores around the lips or mouth.

Arsenicum should be thought of if the herpes sores burn intensely but feel better when warmth is applied. The other typical general symptoms of *Arsenicum* may also be present.

Natrum mur. is indicated when herpes blisters containing a clear liquid develop about the lips, appearing like little pearls. The lips may be cracked. Often the cold sores appear during a fever or cold. Though the sores may be painful, pain is not as characteristic as with other medicines like *Hepar* or *Arsenicum.*

Herpes sores that are painfully sensitive to touch or cold suggest *Hepar.* Pus is likely to form rapidly.

Give *Graphites* if the eruptions ooze a translucent, sticky fluid the color of honey. The individual blisters are likely to be large (pea-sized or larger). They usually itch.

Sepia is considered an important medicine for herpes of both the face and the genitals. Unfortunately, however, there are few distinguishing skin symptoms. If the general symptoms of this medicine (as discussed in the *materia medica* section) match those of the person treated, it should certainly be given. Otherwise we suggest you try it if no other medicine seems to fit or if others haven't helped.

Petroleum is especially indicated for people who have herpes sores in the genital area that are moist and that ooze and itch. The itching may be worse in the open air and better in warmth. In men, the eruption may be on the penis, but more characteristically it is on the scrotum or between the scrotum and thighs. The medicine is equally appropriate for women with genital herpes.

Dulcamara may be helpful when herpes appears on the face or genitals if it seems to have been triggered by exposure to cold or cold, damp weather. The sores are moist, form pus, and may dry to become brown crusts.

Beyond Home Care

See "Beyond Home Care" following "Herpes Zoster."

Herpes Zoster (Shingles)

Herpes zoster ("Shingles") is a skin eruption associated with reactivation of the chicken pox virus. Once a person has had chicken pox, the virus lives on in the nervous system in a dormant state. In some individuals the virus becomes reactivated, travels down a particular nerve, and multiplies at the ends of the nerve in the skin surface. The resulting eruption looks similar to herpes simplex, but the individual blisters are typically bigger, and the overall area of skin involved is also typically larger.

Shingles may erupt on nearly any part of the body, but most commonly it breaks out on the trunk or face. The eruptions are always distributed along the course of the infected nerve. In all but rare cases, only a single nerve is involved, and the rash is confined to one side of the body or one part (a leg, an arm, one side of the face or back). The rash itself usually clears up within a few weeks, but many people have severe pain that lasts for weeks or months because of the irritation of the nerve.

Conventional medical treatment for generally healthy people with herpes zoster is limited to symptom relief, using pain killers and antihistamines that must be taken repeatedly. New antiviral drugs are being tested and are used for patients with reduced immunity. Antidepresssant and anticonvulsant drugs are recommended by conventional practitioners for the pain that lingers after the rash has cleared.

General Home Care

Pressure on the rash may relieve pain and discomfort, and may be applied with snug elastic (Ace) bandage. Cool compresses may also help. Protect the sores with a loose, dry gauze bandage when you are active. You should examine the rash to make sure there has been no secondary bacterial infection (the signs would be pus or redness extending from around the rash).

Homeopathic Medicines

Homeopathic medicines can help the body restore health to the irritated nerves and permanently relieve pain. Untreated, herpes zoster may last three or four weeks, so even when homeopathic treatment is successful, the rash may require seven to ten days to heal, although we have seen better results. You should use homeopathic treatment only if you have no other significant health problems. Select a medicine from the following list and give one dose every twelve hours for thirty-six hours. Stop if you notice any reaction, even after the first or second dose. If no changes are observed after twenty-four hours following the last dose, try another medicine in the same way. Once improvement does begin, repeat the medicine whenever symptoms start to worsen, but no more than twice daily.

Arsenicum is an especially important medicine for people with herpes zoster. The eruption burns intensely, and there is relief in

---

Beyond Home Care

These indications are for herpes simplex and herpes zoster.

Get Medical Care Today:

- if an apparent herpes eruption is located on the face, especially if near the eye;
- if you have any sores on the genitals or develop an eruption after sexual contact, unless you're sure it is a recurrence of herpes you've had before;
- if the rash has lasted longer than a week without improvement;
- if there are signs of secondary bacterial infection—much pus, spreading redness, or swelling. Some pus in the herpes sores is expected, even when there is no significant bacterial problem (see "Beyond Home Care" in the sections on boils and impetigo).

We recommend you be examined the first time you get any eruption you think may be herpes.

See Your Practitioner Soon:

- if you are pregnant and have a rash that may be herpes. Call your practitioner today if you are in the last third of the pregnancy and this is the first outbreak.

warmth and aggravation from cold air or cold applications. The general characteristics of the *Arsenicum* patient may be in evidence. *Rhus tox.* is indicated by intense itching as well as pain. Pea-sized blisters filled with a yellowish but watery fluid appear. Gently rubbing the inflamed areas may give some relief, and lightly moving around also helps.

Lachesis should be considered if the rash is very dark red or especially if it looks bluish or purplish. The eruption is very painful and is extremely sensitive to touch. Typically, *Lachesis* eruptions are worse on the left side of the body.

Ranunculus bulbosus often proves helpful during an attack of shingles, particularly when it involves the chest or back. The pain is severe, especially between the ribs, and is made worse by touch or motion. Breathing deeply or lying on the rash may aggravate the pain.

Mezereum should be considered when there are burning pains or sharp, lightning-like pains, especially when the pains remain after the eruption is gone. The pains are worse while eating, in bed, and from touch. People who need *Mezereum* are chilly and sensitive to cold air.

Iris versicolor may be appropriate if the rash involves the right side of the abdomen or chest. An unusual feature sometimes seen is the appearance of small blisters with dark points. Digestive upsets may accompany the rash.

Apis, Mercurius, Hepar sulph., and *Sulphur* are all sometimes indicated for the person with zoster. Consult the *materia medica* section and the references to these medicines elsewhere in this chapter if none of the above descriptions seem to fit.

Warts

Warts are overgrowths of skin cells triggered by a viral infection. As the body reacts to the virus, regulatory control of cell division is disrupted, and the infected skin cells begin to grow and divide abnormally, building upon themselves till they form the familiar cauliflower shape of a wart.

Warts are caused by a closely related group of viruses. There are several types of warts, including *common warts,* which most often appear on the hands, feet, and face; *venereal warts,* which grow on the genitals, anus, and surrounding areas; *plantar warts,* which form on the soles of the feet; *flat warts,* smooth, barely elevated, oval spots on the face; and *molluscum contagiosum,* smooth, rounded bumps with a central pit, or plug.

Wart viruses are contagious, but some people are extremely susceptible to infection, others very resistent. Children get warts more easily than adults, and venereal warts are more contagious than other types. The ordinary wart virus is so common, there is no way to prevent your exposure to it. You should not be overly concerned about contact with others who have warts.

People who already have them do notice that the warts readily spread to nearby areas, especially if the skin is cut or scraped. Shaving cuts are notorious for "seeding" warts, and a whole crop may grow on the throat of a susceptible man. Children with finger warts may spread the infection by pulling on hangnails or biting their nails.

Warts cause no pain or other symptoms unless they are subjected to pressure or friction. Plantar warts usually cause pain during walking, and warts on the writing fingers of school children may hurt.

Conventional treatment of warts involves applying topical agents that chemically dissolve the warts, destroying them with electricity, or freezing them with liquid nitrogen. Warts are not removed surgically, since the virus can easily spread to cut skin. We recommend that you avoid these suppressive measures at least until you've already tried homeopathic medicines or suggestion treatments.

General Home Care

Warts will disappear sooner or later, and it is fine to leave them alone if they are not causing pain. The best treatment for warts is one that makes the body "take notice" of the virus. Once the body starts to fight the virus, warts shrivel up quickly, often in just a day or two, no matter how long they have been there. The power of suggestion is particularly effective in rousing the body's defenses against the wart virus, and we encourage you to try any safe "ritual" treatment for warts that appeals to you.

Homeopathic Medicines

Homeopathic medicines have had great success helping people throw off wart infections. The placebo effect is of course at work here too, but in our admittedly biased observations we have seen many rapid and dramatic successes with homeopathic medicines, more than we've seen with other treatments. You should use homeopathic treatments for yourself or a family member if the warts are numerous, painful, or if their appearance really bothers you. The person may receive treatment if he has no significant health problems.

The best homeopathic medicine for someone with warts is the constitutional prescription, and it's best to have professional care if it is available. If not, try a medicine from the following list and give a single dose. Allow at least two weeks before trying another medicine.

Causticum symptoms include fleshy warts anywhere, but especially near the fingernails or on the face, and warts with extra growth on stalks above the main part of the wart.

Dulcamara may help with warts on the backs of hands or fingers or on the face. They tend to be large and smooth, flat warts.

Antimonium crudum warts are horny and hardened and have a smooth surface. In our experience this medicine has been consistently helpful to otherwise healthy people with plantar's warts.

Thuja warts may be anywhere on the body and of any type, but those that especially indicate this medicine are on the chin, genitals, or anus. These are often soft warts. They may also be painful or bleeding warts.

Nitric acid is also an important medicine when warts appear on the genitals or anus. There may be warts on the lips (also true of causticum). Soft warts, irregular shapes or irregularities on stalks, great pain, especially sharp, sticking pains, and bleeding warts, especially of the genitals are all symptoms that may indicate this medicine's use.

Ringworm and Related Fungal Infections

"Ringworm" is the common name for a fungal skin infection that results in rough, dry, slightly raised eruptions that occur in usually circular patches. The infected area is slightly reddened. As the eruption gradually enlarges, the central portion begins to heal and clear, while the advancing border remains slightly raised and reddened. This results in the ringlike appearance that gives the infection its name. This is the typical pattern, but ringworm infections sometimes occur without having the clearing in the center or without being circular in outline. Pus does not form, and if the eruption is left alone, it does not become raw or scabby.

Ringworm is known medically as *tinea corporis*. Other related fungi also cause skin infections. *Tinea capitis* is ringworm of the scalp; athlete's foot, jock itch, and fungus infections under the nails are all called *tinea cruris*. A similar skin fungus causes *tinea versicolor*, an infection of the face, trunk, and extremities, consisting of light or fawn-colored, oval, slightly scaly patches that do not tan. Children seem particularly prone to ringworm of the body and scalp, but athlete's foot, jock itch, and tinea versicolor occur in individuals of all ages.

Severe itching is the worst potential symptom of these infections, but often there is no itching at all. There are no serious complications, and all of these fungal infections are only moderately contagious. Even people who have direct contact with the eruptions may not come down with the infection themselves. On the other hand, contact with the lesions, or with clothing, personal articles, or locker-room floors used by infected individuals does spread the fungi. Those with tinea infections should be careful to avoid spreading the germs. If you have athlete's foot, avoid stepping barefoot on locker-room floors.

Conventional medical treatment involves antifungal creams, ointments, powders, or sprays. These topical medications have few side effects, but we still recommend you first allow the body to do its own housecleaning before you resort to conventional treatments.

General Home Care

Ringworm and related fungal infections do eventually clear up if untreated, but you can usually hasten their departure. Simple home measures include keeping the infected area dry and, if possible, exposed to light (this is especially important for jock itch and athlete's foot). Wear clean clothing and socks. Painting the area with vinegar diluted with equal parts of water once or twice a day may help the skin to clear more quickly.

Homeopathic Medicines

People who have ringworm but few other symptoms are difficult to treat with homeopathy, since the skin problem itself usually causes so few symptoms. If there are other problems in addition to the fungus infection, you should receive professional constitutional care. Otherwise, choose a medicine from the following list and give a single dose once a day for three days. Stop if the symptoms change, and allow the healing process to continue on its own. Wait a week before trying a new medicine.

Sepia is probably the most commonly useful medicine for those with simple ringworm infections. The circular, scaly patches are

---

Beyond Home Care

See Your Practitioner Soon:

- if an apparent ringworm eruption lasts longer than a couple of weeks, or if you need help in diagnosis.

dry and brownish or brownish red. There may be itching, which changes to burning after scratching.

Tellurium is indicated when the ringworm is more red than brown. The rings are therefore well marked and prominent. Tiny blisters that itch and release a thin liquid may appear on the rings.

Graphites may help, particularly if the scales are thick or if there is significant oozing. The fluid is usually sticky and honey-colored.

Sulphur may be indicated if the eruption itches a great deal, more so if warmth causes itching. General symptoms of *Sulphur* may be present.

All of the above medicines may be helpful when the ringworm is on the scalp. Two medicines also particularly indicated for ringworm of the scalp are *Calcarea* and *Dulcamara*. Both include thick crusts on the scalp that may be accompanied by swelling of the lymph nodes in the neck and head. *Arsenicum* may also help very dry ringworm with rough scales. Burning and itching are characteristic. There may be a discharge of clear liquid after scratching.

Candida: Yeast Infections

The eruption that results from a *Candida* fungus (known commonly as "yeast") infection is quite different from those triggered by the ringworm, or tinea, fungi. It may start as small, red, raised dots that grow together or spread out from a single infected area. Before long the rash turns into a raised patch or patches of angry red. Between and surrounding the larger patches, small new spots erupt, and the patches spread outward and toward one another. The eruption is dry, as there are no blisters and no pus forms, but the inflamed skin looks raw, and shallow open places may develop.

Candida eruptions tend to spread faster than ringworm infections, at least when they involve areas of the body conducive to growth of the fungus. When the infected person is otherwise healthy, the *Candida* fungus thrives only in warm, dark, moist places on the skin. Common sites are the groin, under the arms, under the breasts, and in skin folds of overweight individuals. Considering these environmental preferences, one can easily see why the *Candida* fungus is so often involved in diaper rashes. The diaper keeps the skin warm and moist, providing the perfect conditions for growth of the organism. In addition, the prolonged contact with the moisture and irritating chemicals of the urine weakens and inflames the skin, allowing the fungus to enter. Even when a diaper rash is initially caused by simple irritation from contact with urine, the *Candida* fungus almost invariably becomes involved within a few days.

The same *Candida* fungus is also involved in vaginal infections (see chapter 9 on women's health) and in the thrush infections of the mouth so common to babies. Thrush is characterized by off-white, elevated patches that may occur anywhere in the mouth. If you scrape off a patch, the underlying lining of the mouth bleeds. Breast-feeding mothers often get *Candida* of the nipples from their children's mouths.

The resistance of the individual is of course a major factor that determines whether or not a person gets a *Candida* infection. Some babies, for instance, never have a problem with diaper rashes, while others get them all the time, in spite of parents' best efforts to keep them clean and dry. Most of the time, even really bad or recurrent *Candida* infections are the result of a specific susceptibility to the particular fungus, and the person is not sickly in any other way. At times, however, frequent or severe *Candida* infections are the first warning of a serious general illness, like diabetes or an immune disorder. Your health practitioner should check such illnesses if you or a family member is prone to severe or recurrent *Candida* infections.

Recently a popular concern has been the possibility of *Candida* infection of the whole system in people with normal immune defenses. Some practitioners and researchers have claimed that undetected systemic *Candida* infections are responsible for a wide range of symptoms and illnesses. Whether this is actually true or not isn't the primary issue. An underlying imbalance or susceptibility must exist to allow any infection to become established, and treating the infecting germs does nothing to restore balance. Constitutional care should be considered for individuals susceptible to infection and to those with recurrent symptoms.

General Home Care

Exposing the affected area to dry air and light usually enables the body to heal the infection quickly. Babies' diapers should be changed frequently and whenever they become wet. Clean and dry the diaper area carefully before rediapering the child, and allow her to stay out of the diapers as much as possible. It may help to paint the affected area with vinegar diluted to half- or quarter-strength (make sure it doesn't sting the raw skin); vinegar retards the growth of this fungus. Apply sparingly either *Calendula* ointment or *Calendula tincture* diluted 3:1 with water to any raw areas a few times a day.

If there is a thrush infection of the mouth, we recommend you rinse the mouth with vinegar diluted 1:1 with water or with quarter-strengh *Calendula tincture.*

Some people find that strictly avoiding sweets helps quickly heal a *Candida* infection. Homeopathic treatment is usually not necessary unless there is a constitutional susceptibility to frequent *Candida* infections.

Nystatin is the conventional drug usually given for *Candida* infections. It is applied directly to the skin and, in severe cases, it is administered orally too. It is fairly safe, but it is rarely necessary if the above recommendations have been followed.

Homeopathic Medicines

If a *Candida* infection is particularly severe and doesn't seem to respond to the simple home-care measures just outlined, try the best-indicated medicine from the following list twice daily for two or three days. Stop as soon as symptoms improve. Wait another day or two before trying another medicine if there is no improvement.

Belladonna is indicated if the skin is bright red and swollen with inflammation but is not raw or oozing.

Chamomilla is probably the correct medicine if a baby with diaper rash also has the marked irritability and other emotional symptoms typical of this medicine.

If the rash burns and itches greatly, *Arsenicum* may help, especially if it is relieved by warmth or if the general symptoms of the medicine are present. The skin may be cracked or raw, and the watery fluid that oozes out is acrid and inflames the skin over which it flows.

As with other skin conditions, *Graphites* is indicated if the rash oozes a sticky, often honey-colored fluid. Raw areas become crusted. On the other hand, the skin may appear simply dry, rough, and cracked.

Hepar should be considered if there is a secondary bacterial infection, and if pimples develop or pus forms in the raw areas. Discharges smell bad. Extreme tenderness of the inflamed parts and relief brought on by warm bathing also indicate *Hepar*.

Severe itching made worse by heat or bathing suggests *Sulphur*. The skin may be rough and dry, or there may be pimples and pus (as with *Hepar* rashes).

For thrush infections of the mouth:

Borax—Probably the best remedy to begin with if symptoms don't clearly indicate another. The child cries when pulled away from the breast because of the pain. There may be raw sores on the mucous membrane (as with *Mercurius*), especially on the tongue. Although there may be increased saliva, dryness of the mouth is more typical. Compared to *Mercurius*, *Borax* has less swelling and bleeding. *Borax* children sometimes have a strong dread of downward motion or falling.

Mercurius—sore and inflamed mouth that smells offensive. There is a great deal of drooling and salivation, the gums are spongy and bleed easily, and there may be white lines on them. The tongue is puffy and flabby and is imprinted by the teeth. It is heavily coated with a black, white, or dirty-yellow color.

Beyond Home Care

See Your Practitioner Soon:

- if you get frequent or severe *Candida* infections;
- if you are not sure of the diagnosis;
- if pus forms (see sections on boils and impetigo);
- if home treatment fails and the infection is severe.

Sulphur—burning and soreness especially during eating. Symptoms are similar to *Mercurius'*, but the gums and tongue are not so spongy and weak. The general symptoms of *Sulphur* may be present.

Hydrastis—a great deal of thick mucus in the mouth and collected on the tongue. The tongue feels as though it had been burned.

Chamomilla—if the emotional symptoms of this medicine are prominent.

Acne

Acne is always a manifestation of an internal imbalance. The bacteria involved are present on everyone's skin, so they alone don't explain the eruption of pimples. Topical and oral antibiotics are effective in killing these bacteria and often reduce the number of eruptions, but of course such treatments do nothing to change the underlying disorder. Other drugs, both topical and internally taken, work by suppressing the physiological mechanisms that produce the acne; from a homeopathic standpoint they are even worse.

We encourage those with mild acne to follow simple measures of cleanliness and good diet—and leave it at that. Those who have more severe cases should seek constitutional homeopathic care before resorting to conventional drugs.

CHAPTER **14**

Accidents and Injuries

Accidents cause far more deaths and serious injuries to children and young adults than all diseases put together. We strongly recommend you give accident prevention high priority in your family's plan for good health.

If someone in your family does suffer from an injury, your first priorities are to apply the proper first-aid measures and to get medical help if necessary. The Red Cross offers first-aid classes in most localities. Every household should have a current, basic first-aid manual such as the Red Cross *First Aid Textbook.* You should also maintain a home first-aid kit (see the Red Cross book for details) as well as a kit of homeopathic first-aid medicines.

The correct homeopathic medicine can complement the standard first-aid measures taken, as it reduces pain and speeds healing remarkably. Even if an injury requires medical care, you can use homeopathy once the injured person's condition is stable.

Homeopathic treatment of injuries is easy compared to that of the various acute diseases with their highly individualized symptoms, as injuries do not require such detailed casetaking. Homeopaths have found that only a small number of medicines need be considered for each type of injury.

Cuts and Scrapes

Cuts (*lacerations*) and scrapes (*abrasions*) are among the most common of life's mishaps.

General Home Care

One of the first priorities is to stop any significant bleeding by applying firm, direct pressure on the wound or the appropriate "pressure point" for that part of the body (see a good first-aid manual for details).

If the wound is minor enough to be cared for at home, cleanse it with soap and water once bleeding has stopped. Be gentle but thorough, and don't leave any dirt in the wound. Cleaning the wound gently with a Water Pik dental appliance is particularly effective for removing tiny bits of debris.

After the wound has been thoroughly cleansed, apply *Calendula* or *Hypericum* externally as indicated later in this section. If the cut is wide, you may need to bring its edges together with a "steri-strips" or a "butterfly" closure before covering it with a gauze bandage. The bandage is needed to protect the cut while it heals. Try to leave the bandage on for at least three days. Take the bandage off by pulling it in the same direction as the cut runs.

Shallow scrapes generally should be allowed to heal without bandages; it may help if you apply one thin layer of *Calendula* ointment just after your initial cleansing of the wound. Do not repeat the application, however. Remember that the scab forming is the body's way of protecting the wound as it heals. Just let if fall off naturally.

Homeopathic Medicines

Calendula, applied topically, promotes granulation of tissues to heal wounds and burns, helps stop bleeding, and inhibits infection. It is used for shallow injuries, such as scrapes and sores. *Calendula* is available in several different preparations.

Calendula tincture is a mixture of the *Calendula* plant juice and alcohol. The tincture is used in the treatment of any wound that breaks the skin. Since the tincture is prepared with alcohol, to prevent stinging, it should be diluted with water, or preferably, sterile normal saline (available in drug stores). Mix 1 part of the tincture with 3–4 parts of water or saline. After cleansing, use a medicine dropper to apply the diluted tincture to the wound. Cover with a bandage and repeat the application three or four times a day.

Calendula lotion is a nonalcoholic solution of the plant juice, glycerin, and water. Like the tincture, it is used for wounds that break the skin, but dilution is not necessary.

Calendula cerate, or *ointment,* is an extract of the plant juice with a petrolatum base and is good for scrapes and for roughened or chapped skin. It is not appropriate for cuts. The cerate should be applied thinly to scraped knees, chapped lips, diaper rashes, and the like.

Beyond Home Care

Get Medical Care Immediately:

- if profuse bleeding occurs, or if there is numbness, tingling, or weakness in or near the wounded part. There is a good chance that important internal structures have been injured;
- for cuts on the chest, back, abdomen, and face, unless they are very shallow. Vital organs and nerves are fairly close to the surface in these areas;
- if the edges of the wound cannot be held together with tape or adhesive bandages, stitches may be required. Stitches should be avoided if possible, since they can cause further injury. Deep, long, or jagged cuts or those over the joints are most likely to need stitching. Facial cuts, except very superficial ones, should usually be stitched to prevent scarring that would affect appearance. Wounds must be stitched soon after the injury occurs, usually within the first eight hours;
- for cuts on the palm or the palm side of the fingers, unless they are very superficial. Such cuts are particularly likely to become infected, and these infections can be severe and spread rapidly;
- if you cannot remove deeply imbedded dirt.

> **Get Medical Care Today:**
>
> - if you notice much redness, swelling, or pus buildup in or around the wound, if there are red streaks extending from around the wound, or if fever has occurred;
> - if the person is not up to date with tetanus shots. Grown-ups only need them every ten years, though severe or dirty wounds may require earlier repetition. Children need a series of shots to maintain immunity. Call your practitioner if you are not sure whether you need a booster immunization.

Calendula oil, prepared from the plant extract in mineral oil, is an alternative to the cerate for rough or chapped skin.

Hypericum tincture may be substituted for or mixed with *Calendula tincture* for cuts that seem to be infected. Dilute it the same way as you would *Calendula tincture.* You may apply it three or four times daily, or you may soak a cotton pad in dilute *Hypericum tincture* and place it over the wound to use as a compress under the bandage. (For the treatment of infected wounds with internal homeopathic medicines, consult the section on "Boils, Abscesses, and Other Skin Infections" in chapter 13 on Skin Problems.)

In conjunction with the appropriate external application, *Hypericum* may be taken orally if cuts are somewhat deep, if there is much pain, or if the cut is hypersensitive to touch. Besides lessening pain, *Hypericum* speeds the healing process. *Hypericum* in potency should also be given if the injuries involve parts of the body that are richly supplied with nerves, such as the fingers, toes, and spine. If there are shooting pains with an injury, *Hypericum* should be considered.

Bruises

A bruise is a superficial injury caused by a blow that does not break the skin. The blow breaks blood vessels and causes black and blue discoloration under the skin.

General Home Care

Apply ice packs to the injured parts for twenty to thirty minutes if the injury is more than mild. This will help reduce swelling and speed the healing process.

Homeopathic Medicines

Arnica is the first medicine to consider for bruises. It helps reduce pain and speeds the absorption of blood under the skin. The more severe the bruise, the more frequently should you take *Arnica*. If the bruise needs treatment but is minor, take *Arnica* two or three times a day. To treat severe bruising, it should be taken every hour or every other hour the first day, and then less frequently the next couple of days. In any case stop after five days.

Ledum should be considered for black eyes or severe bruises that feel cold and numb and that feel better with cold applications. Take the same dosage recommended for *Arnica*.

Ruta is indicated for bruises of the *periosteum*, the membrane that covers the bones. *Ruta* often relieves the pain that follows bruising of the shin, kneecap, or elbow.

Beyond Home Care

See Your Practitioner Soon:

• if you bruise very easily.

Puncture Wounds

A *puncture wound* is one that is deeper than it is wide. Puncture wounds are particularly dangerous for four reasons: (1) they may penetrate deeply into the body; (2) they may push foreign bodies deep into the tissue where the material can be difficult to find and remove; (3) they are difficult to clean and thus more susceptible to infection; (4) they provide a perfect environment for the tetanus germ to thrive and multiply, since this bacteria can only grow in the absence of oxygen.

General Home Care

Clean the wound as thoroughly as you can, using soap and water. Unlike cuts, a puncture wound should be allowed to bleed as long as it can so foreign bodies, dirt, and germs can be carried out of the wound. You should not stop the bleeding unless it is severe or it seems as though some pressure is forcing the blood to squirt from the wound. If, in such cases, there is any chance at all that a foreign body has remained in the wound, carefully apply pressure not directly to the wound, but to the pressure point over the artery of the wounded area (see a good first-aid manual for instructions). Use the pressure point so you don't push a foreign object in deeper, further cutting internal structures.

Soaking the wounded part is advisable, as it keeps the wound open to facilitate the exit of germs and other material, and it brings blood to the area to speed healing. Use warm water and soak the part for 15 to 20 minutes four times a day while there is still pain. If there is any opening in the skin, cover the wound with a sterile gauze bandage and inspect it twice a day for signs of infection.

Homeopathic Medicines

Treat people with deep or painful puncture wounds with both an external remedy and an internal medicine. *Hypericum tincture*, the external remedy, should be diluted with water and applied directly to the wound every half hour or so, and *Ledum, Apis,* or *Hypericum* should be given internally every four to six hours.

Ledum is the most commonly used homeopathic medicine in the treatment of puncture wounds, and you should use it if there are no strong indications for the other medicines. *Ledum* is particularly valuable for punctures when there is redness, swelling, and throbbing pain and when the wound feels cold to touch but is relieved by cold applications. *Ledum* is likely to help puncture wounds even when these specific symptoms are not present.

Apis is indicated for puncture wounds that feel warm or hot with stinging pains and that are made better by cold applications. There is much swelling at the site of the wound.

Hypericum is valuable in the treatment of puncture wounds if there are sharp, shooting pains.

Beyond Home Care

Get Medical Care Immediately:

- for puncture wounds in the abdomen, chest, back, neck, genital region, or head (anywhere except the extremities);
- for particularly deep puncture wounds;
- for puncture wounds in the joints, especially in the knee, since this may cause infection of the joint. Signs of joint infection are redness, swelling and pain in the joint, and inability to move the joint normally.

Get Medical Care Today:

- for puncture wounds in the hands (not the fingers);
- for puncture wounds that remain tender more than two days, that become red or swollen, or that discharge pus;
- if the person is not up to date with his tetanus shots.

Muscle Injuries

Injured muscles result when the muscle group is over-exerted or overextended. Some of the common ways muscles are injured include lifting something too heavy, engaging in vigorous sports you're not accustomed to, and sudden stress on a muscle during a fall or contact sport.

Muscle fibers are actually torn during a muscle injury, disrupting the tissue. Usually the damage is limited to small areas, but extreme stresses can result in tearing of whole sections of the tissue.

Muscle injuries usually take place in large muscle groups (those of the thigh, calf, or bicep, for instance) or in the muscles of the chest and back. Sprains, in contrast, involve the fibrous tissues at or near joints. (See the following section for more information on sprains.)

General Home Care

Though pain is often apparent immediately after an injury, sometimes it isn't that noticeable until a number of hours later. For example, injuries caused by lifting heavy boxes or playing in the yearly football game often first become painful upon waking up the next morning. If you suspect you may have hurt yourself, or if there is pain after an injury, be sure to rest and be cautious about using the possibly injured part. When the part is already injured, it is more susceptible to further damage if used improperly before it's healed completely.

Whether you treat the injury at home or use these measures as first aid on your way to your health practitioner, you should elevate the injured part and apply ice and pressure directly to the area hurt. Cover the ice with a cloth and place it over the injured area, wrapping it firmly with an elastic bandage. If you've wrapped the bandage too tightly, the part may become blue and numb, and the person may complain; if so, rewrap a little less tightly. After half an hour of using the ice-and-pressure treatment, unwrap the bandage to allow blood to circulate to the injured area for fifteen minutes. Repeat the ice-wrapping to unwrapping process for about three hours. If pain has increased substantially by the end of this period, or if pain persists after forty-eight hours, seek medical attention.

After the first twenty-four to forty-eight hours, apply heat with a heating pad or hot water bottle, if heat feels comfortable. A hot bath may help too. Heat brings blood to the area to encourage healing.

We do not recommend the use of liniments containing camphor or other similar medications (Vicks, Heet, Tiger Balm, and other strong-smelling liniments), since camphor tends to neutralize homeopathic medicines. Gentle massage of the painful area is acceptable if it feels good to the injured person and if the injury is mild.

Homeopathic Medicines

After you've taken the appropriate first-aid steps, you may want to use a homeopathic medicine to speed the healing process. Give the internal medicines three or four times a day for a few days, but stop as soon as pain and stiffness improve. *Arnica* is by far the most commonly given homeopathic medicine

---

Beyond Home Care

Get Medical Care Immediately:

- if there is severe pain, distorted appearance of the limb, intense muscle spasm, or collection of blood under the skin;
- if the injured area or the parts beyond it are cold, blue, or numb;
- if the injured person is markedly weak, pale, faint, or sweaty.

Get Medical Care Today:

- if there is continued inability to use the part or if the person cannot bear weight on the injured lower limb;
- if there is a great deal of bruising.

See Your Practitioner Soon:

- if there are recurrent muscle aches without any apparent injury or overexertion.

See Your Homeopath:

- if muscles seem to be injured too easily or frequently. Whether there is weakness of a particular muscle group or excessive vulnerability to injury, constitutional homeopathic care can help strengthen the system. Orthopedic evaluation is also a good idea in such cases. (Also check the "Beyond Home Care" section on strains, sprains, and other injuries to ligaments and tendons as well as the one on fractures.)

in the treatment of people with muscle injuries. It relieves pain, reduces swelling, and speeds healing remarkably. If the injury is slight, we recommend you apply *Arnica oil* externally only, rubbing it into the painful area. If there is significant stiffness or pain, apply *Arnica oil* and give *Arnica* internally as well. Often the pain and discomfort are gone after a good night's sleep. This medicine is often so effective, you may decide the injury was less significant than it was thought to be. Remember that *Arnica* is applicable to muscle injuries, not muscle pain that has resulted from an internal disease process.

Rhus tox. is valuable in treating muscle injuries due to over-exertion. It is also indicated when the most acute symptoms of muscle injury have subsided or when the characteristic *Rhus tox.* modalities are present (worse during initial motion and better during continued motion; see the section on sprains for further information).

Bellis perennis should be considered for deep muscle injuries or injuries to the joints, especially when *Arnica* doesn't seem to be working well enough.

Strains, Sprains, and Other Injuries to Ligaments and Tendons

Joints are surrounded and held together by fibrous tissues: *ligaments,* which connect the bones of one joint to another, and *tendons,* which attach muscles to the bones near joints. A *strain* occurs when a ligament is overstretched, a *sprain* when a ligament is partially torn loose. More severe stress can completely separate the ligament from the bone, resulting in a torn ligament. Similar injuries can occur in tendons.

General Home Care

Strains, sprains and torn ligaments or tendons, like muscle injuries, require rest, ice application, elevation, and firm (but not excessive) pressure on the injured part. These measures apply even if the bone is broken. Immediately after the injury, ice or cold packs applied to the injured part (use as directed in the section on muscle injuries) help reduce the amount of oncoming swelling. After twenty-four to forty-eight hours, warm applications or soaking the injured part in warm or hot water often relieves some of the pain. Gentle, careful massage is sometimes soothing to a mildly injured joint.

Rest is extremely important in protecting the injured joint and facilitating healing. It is crucial to avoid any activity that hurts. Crutches, slings, and splints can help keep the joint relatively motionless while still allowing the person to get around. Elastic (Ace) bandages do not really limit motion so you should not do anything with one on that you wouldn't do without it. The mild pressure and support they provide feel good, though, and they can remind you not to use the weak joint and thereby help prevent further injury.

As the injured tissues heal, begin using the joint slowly and carefully. Ligaments and tendons take longer to heal than tissues like skin and muscle, which are softer and better supplied with blood. Four to six weeks or more may be required. Protecting the joint from sudden motion or stress is required throughout that time.

Homeopathic Medicines

Even if medical care is needed for a joint injury, homeopathic medicines can be very effective in speeding the healing process. Give the remedy every three hours or so during the first two days after the injury, and twice a day for several days after that. Stop as soon as there is significant improvement.

Arnica oil can be applied externally, in addition to the appropriate internal medicine. Rub it into the painful area twice a day.

Rhus tox. is the most common medicine used for strains, sprains, torn ligaments, and tendonitis. It is called the "rusty gate" remedy, since the pains and stiffness are particularly worse during initial motion and become better as the person continues to move and limber up. *Rhus tox.* is especially valuable to people who incur injuries after lifting something or overexerting themselves.

Arnica is indicated when there is considerable swelling, bruising, and inflammation of the soft tissue around the joint. It is a valuable first medicine for many people, even those with torn ligaments, when the swelling is most prominent. Once the swelling and bruising have improved, you should switch to *Rhus tox.* or one of the other medicines to help heal the remaining injury of the fibrous tissue itself.

Bryonia should be considered if the pain is greatly worsened by the slightest motion and continued motion only makes it hurt more. There is swelling of the injured joint, but not so prominently as with *Arnica* injuries.

Ruta is a valuable medicine for tendons or ligaments that have been torn or wrenched. It is generally best used after the most severe initial swelling and pain has begun to decrease. It should

---

Beyond Home Care

Get Medical Care Immediately:

- if there is any obvious distortion, deformity, or instability (wobbling or looseness) of the joint;
- if there is severe pain or massive swelling;
- if it is impossible to straighten the joint;
- if the injured part, or the limb beyond the injury, is cold, blue, or numb, or if the limb beyond the injury can't be used.

Get Medical Care Today:

- if the limb cannot be used or cannot bear any weight within the first twelve hours after the injury;
- if use of the joint or its bearing weight is significantly difficult after seventy-two hours;
- if a child suffers injury to the wrist after falling on an out-stretched hand. Such wrist injuries are common, and fractures of the bones of the wrist are not unusual. They are difficult to detect even with X-rays, and your practitioner may want to see the child again or get a follow-up X-ray just to be sure no bone is broken.

Contact Your Practitioner Soon:

- if symptoms do not steadily improve.

be thought of if *Rhus tox.* has not helped, or if the injured part is neither definitely worse during initial motion nor relieved by continued motion. *Ruta* is often effective for people with tennis elbow.

Ledum is valuable for ankle sprains, particularly when the injured part feels cold or numb and is made better with cold applications.

Dislocated Joints

The bones of a joint may sometimes slip out of position following a fall or blow or after an extremity has been pulled. A rare occurrence, dislocation can cause partial or total loss of function and significant deformity. A common dislocation injury in young children is the partial dislocation of the elbow, which can occur if the child is pulled by the arm. Symptoms of dislocation include swelling, deformity, discoloration, or tenderness of the affected area, along with pain during motion or inability to use the part.

General Home Care

Generally, dislocations should not be treated at home and should receive immediate medical attention. While waiting for help, you should carry out the other home treatments mentioned in the section on strains, sprains, and other injuries of ligaments and tendons.

Homeopathic Medicines

Arnica is a medicine par excellence for dislocated joints. It does *not* take the place of having the dislocated parts put back in place. However, it does allay much of the pain and begins the healing process.

If the person is still experiencing some pain after the first two days, consider giving one of the appropriate medicines listed in the section on strains, sprains, and other injuries to ligaments and tendons.

Beyond Home Care

Get Medical Care Immediately:

• if dislocation is suspected.

Fractures

You can't always tell whether a bone is broken by looking at the injured part. Whenever an injury involves a great deal of pain and tenderness, swelling and bruising, or difficulty moving the injured part, there's a good possibility it's a fracture. An X-ray is usually necessary to make this determination. Resetting of a broken bone is often necessary, for without it the bone may heal in a deformed way.

General Home Care

Initial treatment of any injury in which fracture may have occurred involves rest and ice packs. Apply ice as directed in the section on muscle injuries, using gentle pressure. Since movement of the broken ends of the bone can cut blood vessels or nerves nearby, use a makeshift splint to prevent the injured from moving. Splinting is particularly important if the person must be moved. See the Red Cross or AMA first-aid books for instructions. Initial home treatment of a potential fracture is safe if the guidelines listed in "Beyond Home Care" are carefully followed.

Homeopathic Medicines

Immediately after a possible fracture injury, homeopathic treatment can help minimize pain, swelling, and shock. Give the first medicine—either *Arnica* or *Eupatorium perfoliatum*—every three hours during the first two to three days, but less often as the symptoms improve. Once the fractured bones are reset, time and rest will allow healing to take place, and the correct homeopathic medicine will speed the healing process along.

As with any severe injury, *Arnica* should be the first medicine given, since it is so effective in treating the initial reactions to the trauma, both local and general. Bruising, swelling, and tenderness of the injured area along with a dazed, "shocked" mental state are the characteristic symptoms of this medicine.

If the main symptom of a fracture is pain, and there is not so much bruising, you may try *Eupatorium perfoliatum* during the initial period of recovery.

Once the initial pain and swelling have diminished, give *Symphytum*. *Symphytum*, or comfrey, is the herb that has been known for centuries in Europe as "knitbone" because of its ability to aid the healing of fractures. Give *Symphytum* 6x twice a day for two to three weeks or *Symphytum* 30 once a day for seven to ten days.

Bryonia should be considered for fractured ribs.

Silica is an excellent medicine if small chips have been broken from the bone. Give the 6x potency twice daily for two weeks.

Beyond Home Care

Get Medical Care Immediately:

- if there is obviously a serious injury, a possible neck or back fracture, or if the person is unconscious. Do not move her. Stay with her while someone else goes for medical help. Treat her for shock according to the Red Cross or AMA guidelines while you wait for help to arrive.
- if the possibly fractured part or the limb beyond the injury is bluish, numb, or cold, or if the limb beyond the injury cannot be used;
- if the person feels faint or abnormally thirsty or is sweaty or pale;
- if the injured area is obviously distorted or deformed;
- if the possible fracture involves the thigh or pelvis.

Get Medical Care Today:

- if there is marked bruising or bleeding under the skin in the area of the injury, or if the injury was caused by severe force;
- if the limb cannot be used or cannot bear any weight within the first twelve hours after the injury;
- if there is still significant pain forty-eight hours after the injury, or if use of the joint or its ability to bear weight is significantly difficult after seventy-two hours;
- if a child injures the wrist after falling on an outstretched hand. Such wrist injuries are common, and fractures of the bones of the wrist are not rare. They are difficult to detect even with X-rays, and your practitioner may want to see the child again or get a follow-up X-ray just to be sure no bone was broken.

See Your Practitioner Soon:

- if symptoms do not steadily improve.

Head Injuries

Dr. Spock once said that the child who has never bumped his or her head is being watched too closely. The experience is not an unusual one for adults either. Most of these head injuries are minor and are nothing to worry about. Even if a "goose egg" develops, the injury is usually only a bruise to the skull and scalp. The severity of the injury does not depend on how big the bump is.

General Home Care

Many of the symptoms indicating serious problems do not begin for many hours or sometimes for a couple of days. During this period, unless the injury is just a minor bump on the head, you should check the injured person regularly for the symptoms listed in "Beyond Home Care." Whenever a bad fall or blow to the head has occurred, remember also to check for injuries elsewhere on the body.

Beyond Home Care

Get Medical Care Immediately:

- for any obviously severe injury, or if there is a definite soft area in the bone;
- if there is any loss of consciousness, even momentary, resulting from the blow, or if the person cannot remember the events surrounding the accident;
- if there is diminished mental alertness. Increasing lethargy or unresponsiveness, slurred or difficult speech, abnormally deep sleep, or your own difficulty rousing the person from sleep are danger signs. A person who has sustained a blow to the head should be awakened from sleep every thirty minutes during the first six to eight hours;
- if there has been a seizure or convulsion. During a seizure the person should be placed on his side so he cannot fall or choke on saliva or vomit. Stay with him while someone else gets medical help;
- if there is severe or persistent vomiting. Vomiting once or twice after a head injury is to be expected and does not necessarily indicate severe problems. If there is repeated vomiting, especially after the first few hours, there may be a more serious injury;
- if there is severe or persistent headache. The pain should gradually diminish with time;
- if there is blurred or double vision, other visual disturbance, or difficulty moving the eyes normally;
- if the pupils are of unequal size, unless the person's pupils are normally so;
- if there is difficulty moving all the extremities equally well;
- if there is clear or bloody fluid coming from an ear or nostril;
- if the pulse or breathing is slow, irregular, or weak.

If none of the danger symptoms is present, apply an ice pack to the injured area to minimize swelling.

Homeopathic Medicines

Arnica, once again, is the medicine for treating those with head injuries. Give a dose every three hours for the first couple of days, but give the medicine less often or stop altogether if there is notable improvement.

People who have any chronic or recurrent symptoms that began after a head injury may try a single dose of *Natrum* sulph 200c or 1M. We recommend this treatment only if (1) you only have significant symptoms related to the head injury, and (2) you do not have access to professional homeopathic care.

Burns

Burns can be caused by excessive heat, acid or alkaline substances, or electricity or radiation. When the only apparent damage results in redness of the skin and pain, the injury is a first-degree burn. Burns caused by the sun or brief contact with a hot pan are typical examples of first-degree burns. A second-degree burn causes blistering of the skin as well as redness and pain. When all the layers of skin are burned through and the skin appears deathly white or charred black, a third-degree burn has occurred.

General Home Care

Since burns are the second leading cause of accidental death among children under age four and the third leading cause among older children, prevention of burns is essential. Keep matches and cigarette lighters out of children's reach. Don't have gasoline or other flammables in the house, and if you do, keep them locked up. Install child-proof plugs in electrical sockets. Be sure you never smoke in bed, and have a good smoke-alarm system installed in the house. And finally, keep a working fire extinguisher.

Treatment of first-degree and not-so-extensive, second-degree burns may ordinarily be carried out at home. Conventional treatment of these burns includes immediately applying cold water to the affected part for at least five minutes or until the pain stops. Immersing the burned part in a sink or bucket full of ice water is the best way.

A Band-Aid is not necessary unless the burned part is liable to be bumped or rubbed. Blisters will protect the burn and prevent infection, and thus, if possible, should not be broken. If a blister is large, it should only be broken antiseptically. Most authorities now recommend that the skin of the collapsed blister be removed to prevent infection. The open wound should then be dressed with *Calendula lotion* or dilute *Calendula tincture* as directed in the section on cuts. Change the dressing two or three times a day.

Chemical burns also require immediate treatment. Remove any clothes affected immediately. Most chemical containers have in-

---

Beyond Home Care

Get Medical Care Immediately:

- for any third-degree burn. Do not try to remove charred clothing from the burned tissue. Treat for shock while awaiting medical care.
- for second-degree burns that cover an area larger than the hand or that occur on the face, hands, or genitals. Follow the instructions given for third-degree burns;
- for an electrical burn. Do not use your bare hands to pull the person away from the source of the electrical burn. Use a nonconductive material (a board, mop, wooden chair). Apply mouth-to-mouth resuscitation or CPR as necessary.
- for any radiation burn.

Get Medical Care Today:

- if there is evidence of infection, such as increased swelling and redness around the burn or pus. (See the section on skin infections in chapter 13.)

formation on them about treating burns. Follow their instructions. If the instructions aren't available, wash the chemical off with large amounts of water. Treat the burn as a regular burn after this.

The use of local anesthetic creams or sprays is not recommended for treating burns, since they tend to slow the healing process.

Homeopathic Medicines

Burn injuries can benefit from both external applications and internal medicines. First-degree burns should be treated with topical applications of *Calendula* (*tincture* or *lotion*). *Urtica urens* may be used internally every few hours for pain if needed. Stop whenever improvement continues.

Use topical *Hypericum tincture* for second-degree burns, but be sure to apply it gently so you don't break the blisters. Holding a medicine dropper just over the burn, let the liquid run over the injury. *Cantharis,* or if it isn't available, *Urtica Urens,* may be given internally, according to the directions for urtica urens above. After blisters have popped, *Calendula tincture* diluted with water 1:3 or *Calendula lotion,* when applied two or three times a day under a protective-cotton gauze bandage, can help the sore heal quickly.

For third-degree burns, *Cantharis* should be given internally. Do not use any external applications. With the permission of your health practitioner, you may try *Calendula tincture* (as recommended above) during the latter part of the healing process to reduce the chance of scarring.

Phosphorus, given two or three times daily for several days is the medicine of choice for people with electrical burns.

Shock

Technically, *shock* is the disorder that occurs when blood flow is reduced to below the levels needed to maintain vital functions. Obviously, shock can occur during serious injuries or illnesses that involve loss of blood or other body fluids, but it can also occur during infection, allergic reaction (*anaphylaxis*), or malfunction of the nervous system.

In a sense, every significant injury is accompanied by some

degree of "shock" because the nervous system's acute reaction to the stress of the injury alters blood flow. You should treat any injured person for shock in addition to treating them specifically for injuries. If there is much bleeding, major burns, or a head injury, treatment for shock should be an especially high priority.

Symptoms of shock include general weakness; cold, pale skin; rapid, weak heart rate; reduced alertness; confusion or unconsciousness; and shallow, irregular breathing.

General Home Care

Have the patient lie down with his legs elevated somewhat above the head. Don't bend the legs. Loosen clothing at the neck, chest, and waist. Protect the patient from extremes of warmth or cold. If there is any chance a serious injury has occurred, do not move him. Get emergency help immediately. Let him take sips of fluids only if he is fully conscious and alert; do not give him solid foods.

Homeopathic Medicines

Arnica is almost always the first medicine to give for the general effects of an injury. Whenever there is bruising, swelling, or injury to the head or neck, *Arnica* can help the person maintain strength, and it can promote rapid healing. Once urgent first-aid measures have been taken, give a dose every one-half to two hours the first day if the symptoms are marked. The tiny #10 granules are preferrable; just let them stick to the tongue. Or, dissolve a larger pellet or tablet in a teaspoon of water and limit the dose to a single drop. *Arnica* is also sometimes helpful for the aftereffects of an injury. If

---

Beyond Home Care

Get Medical Care Immediately:

• if shock is suspected.

symptoms of any kind can be dated back to a serious injury, you may try a single dose of *Arnica* 30, 200, or a higher potency, if you don't have access to a professional homeopath.

Heat Exhaustion (Heat Prostration)

Heat exhaustion, also called *heat prostration,* can develop gradually after the body is exposed to hot weather if it loses water and salt through profuse sweating or intake of alcohol. The result is mild shock. Common symptoms of heat exhaustion include tiredness, cold and clammy skin, pallid complexion, headache, nausea and vomiting, dizziness, and muscle cramps. Body temperature may be normal or slightly elevated, and you may notice more rapid pulse and breathing. Blood pressure falls.

General Home Care

Get the person to lie down in a cool, darkened area. Raise the feet and rub his legs to aid circulation. Apply wet cloths to his head and body and fan him. Add half a teaspoon of salt to a glass of water and get him to drink it, repeating this every fifteen to thirty minutes for the first three hours. If fainting or unconsciousness occur, treat for shock immediately, and be sure that extremely high temperature has not developed (if it has see the section on heatstroke). After the patient recovers, be sure he avoids further exposure to heat, for he'll be abnormally sensitive.

Homeopathic Medicines

Veratrum album is the most common medicine prescribed for heat exhaustion. The symptoms are profuse, clammy sweat; great weakness, perhaps even collapse, faintness or actual fainting; extreme coldness of the body, especially of the feet, hands, and face; pallor; nausea; rapid pulse; and general stiffness of the body.

Cuprum metallicum has many symptoms similar to *Veratrum album*'s, but with *Cuprum,* cramping is especially pronounced. Stupor with jerking of the muscles and convulsions may occur.

Beyond Home Care

Get Medical Care Immediately:

- if there is significant dullness or loss of consciousness;
- if the symptoms do not get better within an hour, or if they get worse.

Heatstroke (Sunstroke)

Heatstroke can come on suddenly when the weather is very hot. Its most frequent victims are older individuals and people who exercise in the heat. This is a life-threatening emergency. A failure of the heat-regulating mechanisms of the body results in high fever (104° or higher) and sometimes an inability to perspire. The skin is red, rather than pale, and is hot. Perspiration may be absent, but other times it is profuse. The pulse is fast and forceful. Confusion, stupor, and unconsciousness are common. If conscious, the person may complain of headache, nausea, or visual disturbances and sometimes experiences convulsions.

General Home Care

The body must be cooled immediately. Remove the person's clothing and put her in a cool, shady place. As soon as possible, immerse her in a tub of cold water, and stir the water frequently. If you haven't a tub, apply ice packs to the body. If neither a tub nor ice is available,

Beyond Home Care

- Heatstroke is a medical emergency that requires immediate professional treatment.

sponge the skin with water or alcohol, or spray the person with water. Continuously fan her to further the cooling. Rub the arms and legs vigorously to get the blood flowing again. Make sure breathing is not obstructed.

As soon as the patient's temperature drops to 102° (be sure not to overchill her), dry her off and take her immediately to the nearest emergency room. If you have help, you may be able to transport her while you or others continue the efforts to cool her. If you are alone with the victim, your first priority is to get the temperature down.

After the person recovers from heatstroke, exposure to hot temperatures must be avoided for some time.

Homeopathic Medicines

When treating people who suffer acutely, give the medicine as frequently as every fifteen to thirty minutes the first couple of hours, then diminish it to every hour or every other hour as the person recovers, and stop altogether after twelve to twenty-four hours. Later, constitutional homeopathic treatment from a professional can help reduce abnormal sensitivity to heat.

Belladonna and *Glonoine* are the two most common medicines for individuals suffering the effects of heatstroke. Both cover such heat exposure symptoms as fever, throbbing headache, reddened face, and stupor. Though both medicines tend to be good for individuals with throbbing headaches, *Belladonna* patients tend to have greater burning of the skin than *Glonoine* patients. *Belladonna*'s symptoms are made better by bending the head backward, sitting silently, and keeping the head uncovered, while *Glonoine*'s symptoms are made worse by bending the head backward and applying cold water (which sometimes causes spasms) and better by uncovering and being in the open air.

Insect and Spider Bites and Stings

Human beings usually have the advantage when they encounter other creatures of the earth. But the painful, and sometimes dangerous, bites and stings of insects and other arthropods (insects, spiders, ticks, and mites) serve to remind us that our dominance isn't absolute.

Every bite or sting is accompanied by a local reaction to the venom or the insect's saliva. Ordinarily the temporary pain, itching, and discomfort of a local reaction do not seriously influence a person's health, though some spider bites may cause serious local reactions. In most cases, the inflammation is readily recognized as the organism's effort to localize the infecting venom or saliva to keep it from affecting other parts of the body.

Systemic reactions to bites and stings are rare, but when they do occur, they often need immediate medical attention. The three most common systemic reactions to bites or stings include hives or other skin rashes, wheezing or labored breathing, and fainting or loss of consciousness.

General Home Care

If the insect's stinger has penetrated and remains in the skin, it should be immediately removed by flicking it out with a fingernail. Pulling it straight out sometimes causes additional venom to be injected into the skin. Place a cold application on the stung or bitten part to slow circulation and keep the problem localized.

Homeopathic Medicines

Choose a homeopathic medicine from the following list, and give it every one to three hours. Stop as soon as any substantial improvement is noted, and repeat only if improvement ceases.

Ledum is the medicine most commonly used to treat bites and stings from insects and their kin, and is especially good for bee stings. It helps relieve the redness, swelling, stinging, and pricking pains that accompany a bite or sting. Give *Ledum* routinely unless some other medicine is distinctly indicated. Characteristically, the affected part feels cold yet is relieved by cold applications, but you may still use *Ledum* whether or not this symptom is present. *Ledum* often brings relief even when the swelling involves the whole hand, foot, or limb.

Beyond Home Care

Get Medical Care Immediately:

- if you suspect a bite is from a poisonous spider;
- if there is any difficulty breathing;
- if there is any fainting, confusion, or loss of consciousness;
- if there is swelling in the mouth or throat;
- if there is severe or rapidly spreading swelling;
- if any of the above symptoms have previously occurred after a bite or sting by the same insect.

Apis is indicated if the bite causes marked redness and swelling, especially if the affected part is very hot and the pain is made worse by heat. Use *Apis* if the sensation of hotness is marked or if *Ledum* has not reduced the pain and swelling after four hours. *Apis* is also the medicine to use if hives develop after a bite or sting (*Urtica urens* is an alternative medicine for people with hives after a bite or sting).

Staphysagria is an excellent medicine for children who get mosquito bites that become large and irritating.

Snake Bites

The venom of a poisonous snake contains a highly toxic mixture of enzymes and other proteins that can cause capillary destruction, internal bleeding, paralysis of the nervous system, shock, and death. If you or a family member has been bitten, go to an emergency room immediately.

General Home Care

When treating a person who has been bitten by a poisonous snake, move the person slowly and as little as possible, since vigorous motion can pump the venom through the body more quickly. Ex-

Beyond Home Care

Get Medical Care Immediately:

• if poisonous snake bite is suspected.

citement and strong emotion can also stimulate blood flow, so the person should be reassured. Help him relax by talking slowly and quietly. Remove every piece of jewelry and any clothing that is the slightest bit constricting to the bitten limb. The bitten part should not be moved except when absolutely necessary.

If possible, position the person in such a way that the bitten part is below the level of the heart. Be sure not to give any medication, including aspirin or alcohol. Drugs can cause complications when antivenom medicine is given later in the emergency room.

Additional measures should be taken if you are over thirty minutes from medical care. Tear a broad strip of cloth (two inches wide or more) and wrap it firmly around the bitten area and around the limb. The band must not be too tight; you should be able to place your finger underneath it fairly easily. Since swelling of the extremity continues to spread after the bite occurs, the band should be checked for tightness every ten minutes. Splint the limb so that the joints on either side of the bite are immobile.

Contrary to what most people have heard, tourniquets and immersion in ice do little or nothing to slow the effects of the venom. In fact, their use increases the chance that an amputation will be necessary.

The "cut-and-suck" method for extracting venom should not be used unless you are far from medical care, are certain that the snake was poisonous, and can perform this technique precisely and calmly. Consult a good first-aid manual for details.

Animal and Human Bites

Bites from dogs, other animals, and people are kinds of lacerated or puncture wounds; you should refer to the sections on cuts and punctures for general principles of treatment. These bites can be more easily infected than other wounds. Human bites in particular require early medical attention, since people's mouths are so laden with bacteria. Any laceration of the hand caused by a bite must be cared for professionally. A dog or wild animal that bites must be caught so health officials can be sure it is free of rabies. Squirrels, skunks, and foxes are the most common carriers of rabies. If the animal cannot be apprehended, your health practitioner will consider a variety of factors to decide whether rabies shots should be given.

Beyond Home Care

Get Medical Care Immediately:

- for any animal bite on the hand;
- for any human bite.

Get Medical Care Today:

- if a person is bitten by a wild animal;
- if the animal that bites is not known to be fully immunized against rabies, or if it cannot be caught.

Note: See also the criteria listed in the sections on cuts and puncture wounds.

PART
3

Homeopathic
Materia Medica

The medicines listed here include those most commonly employed in acute care. The psychological and physical general symptoms of each medicine are described, sometimes along with prominent physical symptoms that may accompany any illness for which the medicine is used. When other medicines share the given symptoms, these other medicines are listed in parentheses. For more detail on specific physical symptoms, turn to the appropriate chapters in part 2 of this book.

Although many more homeopathic medicines are used by experienced homeopaths, only the remedies included in the clinical chapters of this book are covered here. There are also a number of medicines included in the clinical chapters that are not listed in part 3. These are not included here, either because the medicine is not known to have significant psychological or physical general symptoms, or because the essential information is covered sufficiently in the clinical section.

The symptoms in these *materia medica* descriptions are condensations intended for use in acute care situations only. Many symptoms that pertain to constitutional treatment are omitted. For more information on medicines listed here, see one or more of the books listed on *materia medica* suggested in part 4.

Aconite*
Monkshood

The symptoms of *Aconite* come on quickly, violently, and intensely. *Aconite* is particularly useful at the beginning of a high fever, during the initial stages of inflammatory conditions, and immediately after

---

See also chapters 3 on fever and influenza, 4 on colds and coughs, 7 on sore throats, 8 on digestive problems, and 14 on accidents and injuries.

the shock of injury or surgery. The symptoms generally begin a short while after exposure to cold or after experiences of sudden fright, anger, or shock.

Because it is normally used at the very onset of an illness, *Aconite* is more often prescribed by laypeople at home than by professional homeopaths. By the time the patient gets to the homeopath, the condition has progressed beyond the *Aconite* stage.

The emotional state of those who need *Aconite* is characterized by acute, panicky fear and anguished restlessness. They may fear death, darkness, crowds, or some unknown, impending evil. In extreme cases they are sure that they will die and may even predict the hour of death. They are very restless, both physically and mentally, and toss about without relief. Their senses are overly acute. Pain drives them to despair, and they are sensitive to light touch, light, and noise. Their sleep is restless; they toss and turn and wake up full of fear, thinking they will die.

Aconite patients may have stomach pain that is made worse by cold drinks (*Arsenicum, Rhus tox.*). During fever, the head may feel hot and full, while the body feels cold.

Although we do not specifically mention *Aconite* in some of the chapters on acute illnesses, this medicine should certainly be considered if the early stages of an earache, a sore throat, a urinary tract infection, or any other illness are marked by the violent onset and general symptoms typical of *Aconite.*

Though both *Aconite* and *Belladonna* cover sudden onset of intense symptoms, people who need *Aconite* are fearful, even panicky, and mentally hyperalert, whereas those who need *Belladonna* are delirious, confused, and less aware of their surroundings. The *Belladonna* patient may fear imaginary things and internal hallucinations, but the fear is not the overriding characteristic as in the *Aconite* case. The *Belladonna* patient is much more likely to be violent and destructive when delirious. Physically, the *Aconite* patient has a flushed, red face, but often this alternates with paleness, or one cheek may be flushed while the other is pale. The *Belladonna* patient's face is consistently flushed. Dilation of the pupils is a symptom more consistent with *Belladonna. Aconite* patients are more likely to experience extreme thirst and usually want plenty of cold water. It is not uncommon for *Belladonna* to be indicated after

Aconite if the latter remedy was given too late or is only partly effective.

Arsenicum is another medicine similar to *Aconite,* and both cover fear and restlessness. But *Aconite* is primarily helpful in the earliest stages of generalized illnesses, those involving the whole system, whereas *Arsenicum* conditions arise later and usually involve a localized infection (sore throat, digestive illness, and so on). *Aconite* patients are generally not afraid to be alone but, instead, are afraid of people or crowds. *Aconite* patients have less general sensitivity to cold or drafts than do *Arsenicum* patients, though the symptoms may have begun after exposure to cold. Both medicines cover extreme thirst, but *Arsenicum* patients may specifically desire frequent sips of water.

What Makes *Aconite* Symptoms

Worse: cold dry wind, rising, night, noise, light, jarring, lying on the painful side

Better: perspiring

*Apis Mellifica**
The Honey Bee

The familiar stinging, burning pain of a bee sting and the hivelike welt it produces are the key symptoms of *Apis* in acute-care situations. Any acute inflammation may call for *Apis* if there is much stinging and burning, marked redness and swelling, and sensitivity of the inflamed part to any form of heat. People with sore throats, hives, conjunctivitis, styes, or insect bites often need this medicine.

Any application of heat makes the pain more intense, and the *Apis* patient gets relief with cold baths or with anything cool applied to the inflamed part. The sore throat is relieved by cold drinks and made worse by warm liquids.

See also chapters 4 on colds and coughs, 5 on childhood illnesses, 7 on sore throats, 9 on women's health, 10 on men's health, 12 on allergies, 13 on skin problems, and 14 on accidents and injuries.

The inflammatory swellings most typical of this medicine have a puffy, water-filled appearance. An inflamed eyelid with a stye looks like a red bag of water, just as if it had been stung by a bee. The inner linings of the eyelids or the surface layers of the eye itself may swell greatly during an eye infection. The throat and palate of the *Apis* patient with a sore throat are red and puffed, and the uvula hangs as though swollen with water.

Those who need *Apis* usually have little thirst, although sometimes they crave milk. The skin is likely to be hot and dry, and it can be sensitive to touch, even when it has no eruptions. Sometimes symptoms initially appear on the right side of the body and then move to the left as they progress.

Sadness and depression can accompany the physical symptoms. The person may weep constantly and without cause. He may be extremely irritable as well, and he may be suspicious and jealous for no apparent reason. He may claim that he is well and doesn't need medical attention even when he is quite ill.

Apis should be considered when illness follows jealousy, fright, rage, or disappointment.

What Makes *Apis* Symptoms

Worse: all forms of heat, hot applications, warm drinks, in a closed or heated room; on the right side, touch, pressure, 3–5 P.M.; after sleep

Better: cool or cold applications, cold baths, open air, uncovering

*Arsenicum Album**
Arsenious Acid; White Arsenic

The distinctive symptoms of *Arsenicum* include great restlessness and fear, severe weakness and exhaustion, intense chilliness, burning pains, and aggravation of the symptoms at night. Whenever this

---

*See also chapters 4 on colds and coughs, 5 on childhood illnesses, 7 on sore throats, 8 on digestive problems, 12 on allergies, and 13 on skin problems.

distinctive group of symptoms appears, *Arsenicum* is the curative medicine, whatever the local symptoms may be.

The *Arsenicum* patient experiences marked weakness and exhaustion, which is often out of proportion compared with the rest of the illness. She becomes exhausted from the slightest exertion. But often this great weakness is accompanied by anxious restlessness. The patient keeps in constant motion until she becomes completely worn out; her agitation makes her toss about in bed or drives her from bed to pace the floor.

Arsenicum patients often feel intense anxiety and fear. A penetrating anxiety about health is common. The patient may be terrified of dying from her illness or from some other catastrophe. Her fears are worse at night, when she also may be tormented by fear of the dark. She is afraid to be alone and must have company for reassurance, else her fears will escalate intolerably. Yet she may not be able to bear being looked at.

She may become possessive about people and things because of her insecurity. She can also be extremely fastidious, and she may be unable to rest if the environment is not meticulously clean.

Burning pains are a key symptom of *Arsenicum.* Any part of the body may burn, but especially the throat, eyes, and stomach. Discharges, like a runny nose or diarrhea, burn and irritate the skin. Most characteristically, all these burning pains are made better by heat. A warm room may help, or the person may want to use a heating pad on a painful infection. Warm drinks relieve burning in the throat and stomach.

In general the *Arsenicum* patient is extremely cold, despite her burning pains. Coldness of any form aggravates her general condition and all her individual symptoms (except the headache, which is made better with cold applications). She craves warmth, which eventually makes her feel much better. Icy coldness of individual parts of the body—forehead, face, chest, knees, hands, or feet—is common.

Most of the symptoms are worse at night, especially between midnight to 2 A.M. The sick person may have trouble falling asleep because of anxiety and restlessness or because of the physical symptoms, such as cough or vomiting, which are worse at night. She sleeps restlessly and has frightening dreams.

Arsenicum patients have a burning thirst, though they may only want sips of water at frequent intervals. They may have a craving for either warm or cold drinks, including milk, though sometimes milk makes them worse.

What Makes *Arsenicum* Symptoms

Worse: coldness of any kind, open air and drafts, night, midnight to 2 A.M., cold food or drink, physical exertion, sea air, right side of the body, fruit

Better: warmth, warm applications, warm food or drinks, the company of others

*Belladonna**
Deadly Nightshade

You can often tell when someone needs *Belladonna* just by looking at him. His face is flushed and the skin is bright red and dry. His eyes are glassy and glaring, and the pupils are dilated. He looks feverish and dull or even stuporous.

Belladonna is generally a medicine for the acute early stages of inflammatory illnesses characterized by high fever and severe pain. *Belladonna* conditions begin suddenly and violently, worsen rapidly, and then leave as abruptly as they started. Fevers, earaches, sore throats, painful menstrual cramps, urinary tract inflammation, and skin infections are some of the most common conditions for which *Belladonna* has been used successfully.

Intense heat, redness, throbbing and swelling are the key symptoms of *Belladonna*. Fever makes the skin so hot it seems to radiate heat. It is said that *Belladonna* is indicated when your fingers remain hot after you have touched the patient's skin. The skin is bright red, maybe even shiny at first, though a dusky flushed complexion may develop with time. Inflamed parts (throat, skin, eardrums) are bright

---

See also chapters 3 on fever and influenza, 4 on colds and coughs, 5 on childhood illnesses, 6 on earaches, 8 on digestive problems, 9 on women's health, 11 on headaches, 13 on skin problems, and 14 on accidents and injuries.

red and swollen but with no pus formation. Swelling develops rapidly during the sudden onset of inflammation, and it causes severe pain. With all the blood brought to the inflamed area, the part burns and throbs intensely.

The *Belladonna* patient experiences heat, throbbing, and a sensation of fullness of the head along with his fever, even while his extremities may be ice-cold. In general, though, he is usually less sensitive to the temperature around him than are those who need medicines such as *Arsenicum, Pulsatilla,* or *Nux vomica.* The skin and mucous membranes are ordinarily dry, but if the sick person is perspiring heavily and other symptoms suggest *Belladonna,* you can still give this medicine. What little mucus, pus, or other discharge there may be is clear and thin. Though they have dry mouths, *Belladonna* patients are generally not that thirsty.

Usually *Belladonna* patients are only dull and tired during the fever. Characteristically, their senses are overly acute, and they may be startled or bothered by noise, touch, light, or jarring motion. In general, however, the patient's attention is inwardly focused, and he is much less responsive to things that happen around him.

Fever often makes the *Belladonna* patient somewhat delirious. In home-care situations this usually does not progress beyond that dull, dazed mentality, or perhaps it leads to some moaning or speaking nonsensically. If the fever is high enough or lasts long enough, however, more severely excited delirium may develop. Scary imaginings and hallucinations may haunt the patient, especially when he closes his eyes. Wild, frightful dreams trouble his sleep. He moans incessantly or his speech wanders or becomes completely unintelligible. He may be startled or may jerk in his sleep or cry out as if he had been shocked. He may even become violent and destructive, breaking things around him, striking at people or imaginary things, or even biting. This sort of behavior suggests serious illness, not a home-care situation, but a dose of *Belladonna* given en route to your health practitioner's office may arrest the crisis.

Belladonna pains are severe, most often of a throbbing or burning type, but the medicine suits any type of pain. The pains are made much worse by sudden jarring motion; even his own walking or someone else touching his bed may jar him intolerably. Sudden touch or pressure increases the pain, but gradually applied pressure may relieve it. Sensations of constriction are common, such as feeling as though a band or strap were wrapped around the head or chest. The person may experience a sensation similar to having a ball inside various parts of the body, especially the throat, bladder, or abdomen. The head, extremities, eyes, or uterus (during menstruation) may feel heavy.

Twitchings of the extremities or other parts of the body may accompany fever. The symptoms may be worse on the right side of the body.

What Makes *Belladonna* Symptoms

Worse: touch, jarring, motion, bright lights, noise, lying on the painful side, rising, letting the affected part hang limply, uncovering the head

Better: lying down, lying on the abdomen

*Bryonia**
Wild Hops

The most distinctive characteristic of *Bryonia* is aggravation from motion. Any type of motion makes the symptoms worse. Walking is intolerable. Simply moving the eyes is unbearable to the *Bryonia* patient with a headache. Deep breathing brings on a coughing spell along with sharp chest pain, and talking can also cause coughing. Swallowing irritates the throat. Even slightly changing the position of some remote part of the body may cause muscular or neuralgic pain. Passive motion, being jarred or carried for instance, also brings on increased pain. When *Bryonia* patients are acutely ill, they want to lie completely still.

Bryonia individuals are also irritable, easily angered, and morose. They don't like to be disturbed and resent being questioned. Adults who need *Bryonia* prefer to be left alone. Sick children are, of course, less likely to want to be completely by themselves, but *Bryonia* children don't want much contact or affection.

---

*See also chapters 3 on fever and influenza, 4 on colds and coughs, 5 on childhood illnesses, 8 on digestive problems, 11 on headaches, 12 on allergies, and 14 on accidents and injuries.

Bryonia patients are likely to be somewhat confused or dull. They may be disinclined to think. Sometimes they feel homesick and say that they want to go home, even when they are already there. They may have business or school affairs on their mind. Even though they are too sick to work, they may talk at length about business or school.

People who need *Bryonia* commonly have headaches, respiratory problems, digestive disorders, or musculoskeletal pains. Motion of any kind may aggravate all of these conditions. On the other hand, firm pressure on painful spots feels good, and lying on the painful part also brings relief.

Many of the *Bryonia* patient's symptoms can get worse after eating. For example, eating aggravates the headache, cough, and abdominal pains. The classical *Bryonia* patient wants plenty of liquids to drink for long intervals. In any case, she is likely to be markedly thirsty. The abdomen becomes painfully distended after eating. The patient may crave milk, sweets, or sour foods. She may be worse after eating fruit, bread, beans, or milk. Although she usually prefers cold drinks, her stomach complaints may be relieved by warm liquids.

Various symptoms of the muscles and joints are likely to appear in the person who needs *Bryonia*. A generalized muscular soreness, which is made worse during motion, commonly accompanies *Bryonia* colds and flus. Joint pains made worse by motion may indicate *Bryonia*, whether they occur during a fever or after an injury.

Dryness is another symptom characteristic of *Bryonia*. The individual often has dry lips, mouth, tongue, and throat. The stools are typically large, hard, and dry and are difficult to expel. The cough is usually dry. The tongue is dry and may have a white, furry appearance.

In general, *Bryonia* patients tend to be worse in heat, in warm rooms, in the sun, and in the summertime and are usually better in cool or open air and also after cold applications. The headache, cough, and muscle and joint pains are worsened by warmth. The *Bryonia* patient may get dizzy in warm rooms and may have trouble falling asleep if the room is stuffy. Cool environments and open air may help relieve anxiety and confusion. Some complaints begin after exposure to cold, however.

The symptoms of people who need *Bryonia* develop somewhat

slowly, as compared with the rapid onset of symptoms occurring when *Aconite* or *Belladonna* is indicated. Many of the pains are worse on the right side of the body.

What Makes *Bryonia* Symptoms

Worse: motion, exertion, jarring, rising, becoming heated, warm rooms, the sun; eating, evening or night, cold (sometimes).

Better: rest, lying still, firm pressure, lying on the painful side, lying down, cold drinks (except when these are stomach complaints), cool rooms, open air

Calcarea Carbonica*
(Carbonate of Lime)

Calcarea carb. is sometimes used during acute conditions, though it is more commonly given as a constitutional medicine. We give instructions for its use in the sections on vaginitis in chapter 9 and skin infections in chapter 13.

People who need *Calcarea carbonica* are physically and mentally weak. They are easily tired and tend to sweat from the slightest exertion. Most commonly, *Calcarea carbonica* is given to people who are plump and fair skinned, have flabby muscle tone, and are prone to swollen lymph nodes. These individuals have strong chills and difficulty keeping warm. They are averse to cold, open air, which seems to go right through them. Exposure to damp, cold weather is aggravating, and an acute illness may develop after being out in a rain.

Calcarea carbonica patients tend to sweat easily. Perspiration of isolated parts of the body is common. The head often perspires during sleep, usually shortly after falling asleep. They may also sweat on the abdomen, upper torso, genitalia, feet, or palms. Perspiration, discharges, and stools often smell sour.

A strong craving for eggs is a classic symptom of those who need *Calcarea carbonica,* but they may also crave raw potatoes, milk, sweets, salt, and indigestible items such as dirt or chalk. On

---

Sulphur should not be given immediately after *Calcerea carb.*

the other hand, they may be averse to milk or meat. They are thirsty, usually for cold or iced drinks.

Calcarea carbonica patients are often passive and complacent people, but they may become surprisingly stubborn if asked to do something they don't want to. They may be slow to comprehend things and have great difficulty with mental effort. They may be afraid of the dark, of being alone, of being ill, or of going crazy.

What make *Calcarea Carbonica* Symptoms

Worse: cold, damp weather, exertion, fright

Better: warmth, lying down

(see chapters 9 on women's health and 13 on skin problems)

Chamomilla*
German Chamomile

Chamomilla patients are cross and irascible, probably the most irritable among the homeopathic-remedy types. Children are particularly given to the open displays of irritability and discontent so typical of *Chamomilla,* so they are given this medicine more often than adults. Nothing pleases the *Chamomilla* patient, and everything seems to bother him. He demands to have something but, when he gets it, he rejects what he so urgently desired and becomes even more upset. He is stubbornly disagreeable and refuses to do anything asked of him. His irritability increases until a screaming tantrum ensues, and a *Chamomilla* child may strike out at anyone within range during one of these fits. He hates to be touched, spoken to, or even looked at, and he bursts into renewed screaming if these attentions are offered. He is extremely sensitive to pain and screams as he suffers it.

Chamomilla people are inconsolable. Soothing words and affectionate touch don't calm them and are likely to make them even more upset. The only thing that may help a *Chamomilla* child feel

---

*See also chapters 5 on childhood illnesses, 6 on earaches, 9 on women's health, 12 on allergies, and 13 on skin problems.

better is being carried about or rocked. He may fall asleep in your arms and then start fussing again as soon as you stop the motion.

The head, face, and feet are especially hot. Often one cheek is hot and red while the other is cold and pale. In spite of the internal warmth, becoming cold is eventually aggravating. These people are generally very thirsty, especially for cold water. Sometimes a sense of numbness accompanies the pains.

What Makes *Chamomilla* Symptoms

Worse: warmth of the bed, anger, night, touch, lying down, lying on the painless side, eating, milk, warm food, open air, wind, cold

Better: being carried, passive motion (such as being rocked), fasting, perspiring, cold applications

*Ferrum Phosphoricum**
Phosphate of Iron

Ferrum phos. is indicated in the first stages of various inflammatory conditions. People who need *Ferrum phos.* have symptoms similar to those of *Aconite* and *Belladonna;* however, the onset of the symptoms of *Ferrum phos.* may not be as rapid or violent. *Ferrum phos.* is most commonly prescribed for people with fever, colds and other viral illnesses, and earaches. It should be chosen when the person doesn't have clear, distinguishing symptoms that would indicate another medicine.

The *Ferrum phos.* patient is flushed and hot with the fever. Classically, there is well-defined, circular redness on the cheeks (usually the entire *Belladonna* face is flushed). She may be sensitive to cold and cold air. She is tired and easily exhausted by physical exertion, and sometimes her illnesses begin after overexertion. She may have a tendency to bleed easily. There may be bright red blood coming from the nose or gums at the onset of a feverish illness, or a dry cough may bring up a little blood-streaked mucus.

Ferrum phos. patients are more alert than those who need *Bel-*

---

*See also chapters 3 on Fevers and Influenza, 4 on colds and coughs, 5 on childhood illnesses, and 6 on earaches.

ladonna, less anguished and fearful than *Aconite* patients. They pay attention to what is going on about them, and even during a high fever follow everything happening in the room with their eyes. Sometimes there is a tendency toward loquacity and mirth. They'll joke and chat as though they weren't ill. The fever can make it difficult for them to concentrate, and sometimes they become forgetful, dull, and indifferent as they tire. These symptoms are like those of *Phosphorus,* but *Phosphorus* is more useful later in the course of an illness and has many other individual symptoms.

What Makes *Ferrum Phos.* Symptoms

Worse: cold, night, exertion, standing

Better: gentle motion

*Gelsemium**
Yellow Jasmine

Drowsiness and mental and physical weakness are the prominent symptoms of the *Gelsemium* patient. The body feels heavy and tired. The patient dreads movement, not because it's painful, but because it's just too much effort. The limbs in particular feel heavy, and there is a general tiredness of the whole body. Sometimes there is weakness of individual parts of the body. The eyelids may feel heavy and droop noticeably, and the face looks sleepy and weary. The limbs are weak and heavy, and the legs tire easily from walking or other exertion.

The mental weakness of the person with a *Gelsemium* illness corresponds to this physical condition. The mind is sluggish, and the person becomes dull, forgetful, and indifferent. She doesn't want to be spoken to and just wants to be left alone in a quiet room. She is really too tired to be irritable.

The *Gelsemium* person with a flu or fever often feels achy all over. There may be stiffness of the neck and upper back. Headache may accompany the symptoms, classically beginning in the neck

---

See also chapters 3 on fever and influenza, 4 on colds and coughs, 5 on childhood illnesses, and 11 on headaches.

and back of the head and extending to the forehead or the entire head. She may experience temporary relief of her symptoms after urinating.

Gelsemium patients often feel chills running up and down the back. They want heat in general, though exposure to the sun may bring on headache. They usually experience little or no thirst. The face may be flushed a dusky, red color.

Anticipation, nervousness, and similar emotions may bring on the symptoms. A *Gelsemium* condition may begin, for instance, because of anticipation of an examination or public performance or after receiving bad news.

What makes *Gelsemium* Symptoms

Worse: anticipatory anxiety, bad news

Better: perspiration, urination

Hepar Sulphuricum*
Hahnemann's Calcium Sulphide†

Physical hypersensitivity and mental irritability characterize those who need *Hepar sulph.* These people are exquisitely sensitive to touch, cold, and pain. Any infected part (such as a boil, stye, or swollen gland) is extremely tender to touch, and the slightest pressure causes sharp pain—as though a splinter or bit of glass were pushing into the affected part. There is a sensation similar to having a splinter or fishbone caught in the throat, and the pain increases upon swallowing.

Hepar patients are so cold the slightest exposure causes chills. Even a hand or foot's sticking out of the blankets may bring on symptoms. Cold air or applications to an infected area make the pain of the inflammation much worse. Dry, cold air may be the

---

See also chapters 4 on colds and coughs, 6 on earaches, 7 on sore throats, and 13 on skin problems.

†Hahnemann developed this medicine by burning a mixture made of the inner layer of oyster shells (a source of calcium carbonate) and flowers of sulphur.

least tolerable. The *Hepar* patient is overly sensitive to pain in general, and pain may make him faint.

Hepar patients are irritable, impatient, and discontented. Everything bothers them, nothing pleases. They are cross and easily angered and may pick fights for no apparent reason. They may have sudden violent impulses, and at times their anger can get out of control. *Hepar* children, however, are somewhat less apt to hit or scream than children who need *Chamomilla.*

The *Hepar* patient commonly has an offensive or sour smell. His sweat, stool, and discharges also smell sour or offensive. Discharges from the nose, pus from boils, and phlegm that is coughed up are profuse and of a thick, yellow, or cheesy character.

The *Hepar* patient loves vinegar, pickles, and other sour foods, as well as spices and strong-tasting foods. He may dislike fats. He may be more thirsty than usual.

What Makes *Hepar* Symptoms

Worse: cold, a single part becoming cold, uncovering, lying on the painful side, pressure, night, dry weather, motion, exertion, tight clothing

Better: warmth, hot applications, wet weather, lying on the painless side

*Ignatia**
St. Ignatius Bean

Although we have recommended *Ignatia* in only two of the chapters dealing with acute care, we include it in this *materia medica* section because of its unique applicability to conditions brought on by acute emotional stress. Whether the symptoms represent disordered nervous system function or the body's response to an infectious illness, *Ignatia* may be the curative medicine if the condition was precipitated by grief, fear, anger, embarrassment, or a scolding.

---

*See also chapters 5 on childhood illnesses and 14 on accidents and injuries.

The *Ignatia* patient usually tries to avoid really breaking down in front of others, but she is given to frequent, loud sighs that betray her inner anguish. Though some *Ignatia* patients never cry, more often, when they are alone, break into involuntary, wracking sobs, perhaps punctuated with spasmodic laughter. The patient feels worse when consoled. She is likely to be inordinately sensitive to reprimand, yet she will often inflict severe self-criticism if she doesn't do something right.

Because of her emotional upset, the *Ignatia* patient is often unable to sleep well. Feeling a lump in the throat is common among emotionally distraught people, and this is characteristic of *Ignatia* as well.

Seemingly contradictory symptoms are distinctive of *Ignatia*. Nausea may be made better by eating, while eating may make hunger more intense. Simple fruits cause indigestion, and heavier foods may be more easily tolerated. Ordinary foods may be repugnant to the *Ignatia* patient, and she may crave indigestible things instead. She may want to be uncovered and to drink when she is cold, just as she may be thirstless during the height of a fever. A roaring noise in the ears may get better when she hears music.

The *Ignatia* patient often craves fruit, although it may cause indigestion. She may jerk and twitch out of nervousness. The senses may be overly acute. Sometimes only one cheek is flushed (also a sometime symptom of *Chamomilla, Nux vomica,* and *Pulsatilla*).

If you decide that *Ignatia* should be given during an acute emotional crisis, give a single dose of the 30x or 30c potency and observe the results for six to eight hours. If the symptoms are unchanged, you may repeat the dose one more time, but if there is still no result, try to find another medicine that fits the symptoms. If *Ignatia* seems to help, repeat it only when the symptoms have grown decidedly worse, and do so no more than twice a day for three days.

What Makes *Ignatia* Symptoms

Worse: suppressing grief or other emotions, consolation, tobacco smoke, pressure on the painless side

Better: eating, lying on the painful side

Kali Bichromium*
Bichromate of Potash

Thick, stringy discharges from mucous membranes are the most distinctive symptoms of those who need *Kali bichromium*. Although many other homeopathic medicines also cover the thick, yellow or green discharges that are typical of *Kali bi.*, a marked sticky, gluey quality is more characteristic of this medicine than of any other. A discharge from the nose, for instance, tends to adhere to the nasal passages and throat and may be so gelatinous that it can be pulled away in stringy lengths (described in the older homeopathic literature as "ropy"). Sometimes the material is discharged in nearly solid globs. *Kali bi.* should be considered whenever discharges of this character are found, whether they come from eyes, ears, nose, or throat.

Other characteristics of *Kali bi.* are symptoms that come and go suddenly and pains that are limited to small parts of the body or that wander from place to place. Commonly, joint pains alternate with digestive problems, diarrhea, or respiratory difficulties.

Kali bi. patients generally get cold easily, but they feel worse in hot weather. These temperature reactions are not as marked as those associated with other medicines we've discussed. The patient in general, and especially his cough, is often worse between 2 A.M. to 3 A.M.

Psychologically, those who need *Kali bi.* tend to be low-spirited, ill-humored, irritable, and indifferent. They are often listless with a great disinclination for mental or physical labor.

Since the strong symptoms are localized "particulars," and since the general symptoms of *Kali bi.* are not well marked, look first for medicines that match any strong general symptoms of the illness before you give *Kali bi.* When a thick, stringy discharge is a prominent symptom, *Pulsatilla* may be indicated if the person is weepy, thirstless, and uncomfortable in warm rooms. *Mercurius* may better suit the patient who is more irritable and thirsty, and is sweaty, is

---

See also chapters 4 on colds and coughs, 5 on childhood illnesses, and 10 on men's health.

bothered by both heat and cold. Use *Kali bi.* if your first choice hasn't helped or if the only striking aspect of the illness is the thickness and stringiness of the discharge.

What Makes *Kali Bi.* Symptoms

Worse: cold, hot weather, 2–3 A.M., undressing

*Lachesis**
Venom from the Bushmaster or Surucucu Snake

Symptoms that are worse upon waking, during sleep, on the left side of the body—along with a unique, "volcanic," mental state—are the primary indications for *Lachesis.* Acute home-care situations in which *Lachesis* is most commonly useful include sore throats, boils and abscesses, and menstrual pain.

Whenever the symptoms of any of these conditions are most intense upon first waking or during sleep, *Lachesis* may be the correct medicine. In fact, people who need *Lachesis* may dread going to sleep, because they anticipate the increased suffering they must endure when they awake. Pain or inflammation that is much worse on the left side of the body, or that begins on the left and moves to the right, is equally characteristic.

The psychological state of the *Lachesis* person has been described as "volcanic." The individual is loquacious, jealous, and suspicious. Excitability and a vivid imagination are typical, and the patient talks nonstop, jumping from one idea to another, sometimes even before finishing his sentence. Unwarranted suspicions and jealousies may arise, and he may believe that others are conspiring against him or that his lover has been unfaithful. Sadness that comes with the morning, especially upon waking, is also a common *Lachesis* symptom.

The sensory system is hyperacute. A classic *Lachesis* symptom is inability to tolerate the pressure of clothing, especially around

---

See also chapters 4 on colds and coughs, 7 on sore throats, 9 on women's health, and 13 on skin problems.

the throat or waist. Even the slightest contact with clothing can be extremely distressing; sometimes the pressure of the blankets aggravates the bedridden *Lachesis* patient. The eyes are sensitive to light, noise is irritating, and light touch is aggravating, though firm pressure may be comforting.

Lachesis patients usually crave open air, so they may open windows even in cold weather. They prefer cool temperatures and want few clothes or covers. Extremes of either heat or cold may cause weakness.

Inflamed areas, whether in the throat, on the skin, or elsewhere, have a dark bluish or purplish appearance. Similarly, the face may look somewhat purplish during the fever or other acute illness.

What Makes *Lachesis* Symptoms

Worse: sleep, waking, touch, pressure, clothing, heat, warmth of the sun, warm rooms, lying down

*Lycopodium**†
Club Moss

Lycopodium is a frequently used medicine in a wide variety of both acute and chronic illnesses. Though you should not attempt to treat chronic conditions at home, *Lycopodium* may be the indicated medicine during home-care situations involving earaches, sore throats, digestive conditions, and urinary tract problems.

Several key general symptoms of *Lycopodium* indicate its use no matter what the specific problem is. Conditions that are definitely worse on the right side, or that begin on the right and then move to the left, strongly suggest *Lycopodium*. The symptoms are often worse between the hours of 4 and 8 P.M. Craving sweets is also characteristic, as is desiring warm drinks which relieve symptoms such as cough, sore throat, or stomach discomfort.

---

*See also chapters 6 on earaches, 7 on sore throats, 8 on digestive problems, and 13 on skin problems.

†*Lycopodium* should not be given immediately after *Sulphur.*

Lycopodium patients are particularly prone to disorders of the digestive system, most often suffering intestinal gas and bloating, along with whatever other symptoms they may have. The distension and gas are worse after eating, and the abdomen is sensitive to the pressure of clothing. The appetite is confused. The *Lycopodium* patient may feel hungry sitting down to a meal, but then a bite or two makes him full. Or he may have a ravenous appetite soon after a big meal (a symptom shared with *Phosphorus*). Sometimes intense hunger wakes the *Lycopodium* patient from sleep, and he may get a headache if he doesn't eat. *Lycopodium* patients tend to be averse to meat as well as generally aggravated after eating oysters, onions, cabbage, or milk.

Lycopodium patients may be warm or chilly, though they usually desire open air and dislike warm rooms. Occasionally one foot is hot while the other is cold. Though they prefer warm drinks, they often have little thirst.

The *Lycopodium* psychology is characterized by insecurity and cowardice. The person becomes anxious and doubts his ability to perform new or challenging tasks. He is especially nervous in social situations and worries about what people think of him. He fears rejection and may think that he is being observed critically. He often tries to hide his insecurity by bluff and bravado, and he may resort to domineering behavior, especially over those younger, weaker, or less intelligent than he. He may not like the company of others, but he can also be afraid to be alone; classically, the *Lycopodium* patient wants to know that someone is nearby but not in the same room.

The *Lycopodium* patient can also be afraid of the dark, of crowds, and of death. Often his anxieties are felt in his stomach. He may be cross and peevish, especially when he first wakes in the morning. Fright, anger, or embarrassment may bring on his illness.

What Makes *Lycopodium* Symptoms

Worse: 4–8 P.M., on waking, warm rooms, eating, pressure of clothing, onions, oysters, cabbage, fruit, milk, cold food or drink

Better: warm food or drink, midnight and later hours, cool or open air, uncovering the head

*Mercurius Vivus and Mercurius Solubilis**
Mercury, the Chemical Element (Quicksilver)

Mercurius vivus, the simple elemental form of mercury, and *Mercurius solubilis,* a soluble preparation of mercury created by Hahnemann, are considered essentially identical medicines by homeopathic authorities. They are used on the basis of the same indications, though the chemical compositions of the two remedies differ.

Mercurius is most likely to be required during acute conditions characterized by marked inflammation of the skin and mucous membranes along with pus formation and perhaps raw, open areas. Examples of these conditions include eye infections with discharges of thick pus; bacterial ear infections with pus buildup behind the eardrum; sore throats with much pain, pus formation, and even open sore spots; urinary infections; and skin infections such as boils and herpes.

In these conditions and others, the person's whole illness follows the distinct pattern of *Mercurius* general symptoms. Although there are times the decision to give *Mercurius* may be based on the particular symptoms alone, you can be sure of your choice if the key general symptoms of the medicine are present. These include: heavy perspiration that often makes the patient feel worse; foul-odored perspiration, breath, and entire body; much salivation, so much that when the patient drools he gets his pillow wet; and aggravation of the symptoms at night, often beginning after sunset.

Mercurius patients, in fact, are aggravated by almost every environmental influence and are comfortable only over a narrow range of conditions. Like a mercury thermometer, they are very sensitive to temperature, and they are bothered whenever it gets even slightly too hot or too cold. They are bothered by open air and drafts, but warm air or a warm bed also makes them feel worse.

Trembling is another general *Mercurius* symptom. The hands,

See also chapters 4 on colds and coughs, 5 on childhood illnesses, 6 on earaches, 7 on sore throats, 8 on digestive problems, 9 on women's health, 10 on men's health, and 13 on skin problems.

tongue, all the limbs, or any other part of the body may tremble or jerk visibly, especially when an effort is made to use them. The *Mercurius* patient is generally weak and tires easily with exertion. The vital responses of the body are weak and slow, and infected tissues are slow to heal and look unhealthy.

On the mental and emotional level, there may be an undirected agitation, restlessness, and hurriedness, along with rapid talking and rushing to get things done. There is an inability to concentrate, which results in impulsiveness as ideas come to mind. At times these impulses can be violent; past *Mercurius* patients have been seized with impulses to commit suicide or murder. The mind is generally dull and sluggish, so the patient may take a long time to answer questions.

Whatever the specific condition afflicting him, the *Mercurius* patient is likely to have prominently swollen lymph nodes as a result of the inflammation. In addition to the salivation and drooling, inflammation and soreness of the mouth is typical, and there is often a metallic taste there as well. The gums are swollen and spongy, and blood oozes from them when they are touched or during eating. The tongue is puffed up and flabby and shows imprints of the teeth.

Often *Mercurius* patients are averse to sweets, meat, fats, or butter, though sometimes they crave buttered bread. They can be thirsty, and they may well have a craving for cold drinks.

What Makes *Mercurius* Symptoms

Worse: heat, cold, dampness, warm air or warmth of the bed, open air, sunset to sunrise, sweating, sweets, motion, lying on the right side

Better: moderate temperature

*Natrum Muriaticum**
Sodium Chloride (Table Salt)

See also chapters 4 on colds and coughs, 10 on men's health, and 13 on skin problems.

During an acute illness, *Natrum muriaticum* may be indicated by the specific physical symptoms, even if its general symptoms are not evident. If the psychological or physical general symptoms are present, your choice of this medicine is the more certain.

Natrum muriaticum patients often become ill after experiencing some type of emotional trauma. They have particular difficulty dealing with loss or rejection—the breakup of a relationship or the death of a loved one—which may weaken their system and precipitate an illness. They also tend to get symptoms after being reprimanded. Although these people are emotionally sensitive and their feelings are easily hurt, they have difficulty expressing their emotions. They hold in grief, anger, disappointment, or frustration and rarely weep in front of others. When alone, however, they may break down and weep loudly. The *Natrum muriaticum* patient may avoid intimacy to prevent being hurt. He wants to be alone when ill, and he feels uncomfortable and irritable when others try to console him.

Sudden noises, like the ringing of a telephone or the slamming of a door, may unduly startle the *Natrum muriaticum* patient, and he may even feel weak and ill afterward. He may be deeply affected by music.

The person tends to be physically warm and is bothered by heat. He is often sensitive to the sun, which may cause exhaustion or a headache. He feels better in the open air or perhaps after a cold bath.

The classic *Natrum muriaticum* patient craves salt, salty foods, and possibly bread. Sometimes, however, he is averse to bread or salt, and more often will dislike fats or slimy foods.

Dryness of the skin and mucous membranes is common, but the face and the hairy parts of the body may be oily. Stools are also often dry and become hard and difficult to expel.

What Makes *Natrum Muriaticum* Symptoms

Worse: grief, heat, sun, 10 A.M., noise, music

Better: open air, cold bathing, fasting

Nux Vomica*
Seeds of the Poison-Nut Tree

Nux patients are irritable, quick-tempered individuals who get sick by overeating, indulging in alcohol or drugs, or doing too much mental work. Although you may decide to use *Nux* during an acute illness on the basis of the particular symptoms alone, if these key general attributes of the *Nux* patient are present, your choice is confirmed.

Impatient irritability marks the *Nux* patient's psychology. He is prone to argue and may start quarrels over any imagined offense. He feels hurried and driven to accomplish things. He can't stand to wait for others. He is likely to be critical and quick to reproach anyone who doesn't live up to his demanding standards. He can snap sharply when irritated. Or instead, he may try to keep his annoyance to himself, but his displeasure shows in his blunt, undiplomatic language and the frown on his face. He prefers to be left alone and hates having to depend on others less capable than he. He hates to be questioned.

The *Nux* patient is fastidious and fussy over little things, and he may have a compulsion to arrange his environment according to his own precise sense of order. His nervous system is overly sensitive. Slight noises, such as the sound of people talking or even the sound of footsteps, drive him to distraction, and he can't stand bright lights or unpleasant odors.

Nux patients are particularly chilly and are made worse by cold weather, especially dry, cold weather (a symptom shared with *Hepar*). When they are feverish, they get severe chills and cannot warm themselves even when sitting by a heater. During the fever they cannot stand to uncover or undress, and any slight movement of the covers sets off a new wave of chills.

Sleep is difficult for the *Nux* patient. He may have trouble getting to sleep because of an overactive mind or because he notices every little noise. Or he may wake early in the morning and be unable to get back to sleep. He is especially irritable when awakened from sleep or a nap.

See also chapters 3 on fever and influenzas, 4 on colds and coughs, 8 on digestive problems, 11 on headaches, and 12 on allergies.

The digestive system is often a weak area for the *Nux* patient. Even if the main problem is a respiratory illness or involves some other system, it is usually accompanied by some of the typical *Nux* digestive disorders. The digestive system is generally weak and the *Nux* patient is intolerant of many foods. Indigestion, heartburn, nausea, fullness and bloating of the abdomen, gas, and constipation or diarrhea may beset the *Nux* patient in any combination.

A craving for stimulants, alcohol, and other drugs is common to *Nux* patients. Very often overindulgence in drugs brings on the symptoms. Because it so closely covers the common symptoms of an alcoholic hangover, including the typical headache and digestive distress, *Nux* is a most effective medicine for people with that condition. We recommend, if you take it under those circumstances, do so only very occasionally.

Nux patients are also known to crave fats, spicy foods, and milk. They can be quite thirsty, though drinking may cause bloating of the abdomen.

Other characteristic *Nux* symptoms include a tendency toward twitchings or spasms of various muscles (including muscles of the eyelids, limbs, back, and abdominal wall); headaches; and lower back pain that is particularly aggravated by turning over in bed.

What Makes *Nux Vomica* Symptoms

Worse: anger, mental exertion, morning, cold, eating or overeating, spices, rich food, stimulants, narcotics, alcohol

Better: resting, evening

*Phosphorus**
The Chemical Element

Phosphorus is a deep-acting medicine that is rarely used during the beginning of an illness. In acute care it is most commonly given for coughs and digestive problems. The physical symptoms typical of *Phosphorus* patients include a restless, overexcited state that

---

*See also chapters 4 on colds and coughs, 8 on digestive problems, and 14 on accidents and injuries.

leads to weakness and exhaustion, chilliness combined with a thirst for cold drinks, and burning pains.

Equally characteristic are the mental symptoms. People who need *Phosphorus* are cheerful, friendly, open, and impressionable. They are bright and their perceptions are quick. Even during acute illnesses *Phosphorus* patients are likely to be much more alert and interested in their surroundings than you might expect. They have active imaginations. They are expressive and animated. They are overdramatic when demonstrating their emotions. Their senses are acute; they are bothered by light and noise and are easily startled. They may be intuitive and even psychic. Nervousness and fear are quick to develop in their active, impressionable minds. They may fear the dark, thunder, imaginary things, illness, or death. Sometimes there is just a sense that something bad will happen.

Phosphorus patients are sociable and crave company. They are often fearful when they are alone. They seek sympathy and attention and feel better when they get it but, compared to *Pulsatilla* patients, they more often want to actively return affection. They can get frightened or upset easily, but reassuring words or distractions help them quickly forget their troubles.

Although they are enthusiastic, *Phosphorus* patients lack stamina and easily become tired both mentally and physically. At first, the patient may hardly seem ill, with energy and vitality unusual for a sick person. He may be over excited and physically restless, and he may begin many projects. But excitement gives way to exhaustion, depression, or irritability, and the projects are left unfinished.

Phosphorus patients usually feel cold, and their symptoms are made worse by cold and better by heat, though sometimes the opposite is true. They are sensitive to sudden changes of weather. Open air may either aggravate or relieve the condition.

Phosphorus patients crave salt, spicy foods, and ice cream (which relieves stomach pain). The patients are generally thirsty for plenty of cold or iced drinks, though these may cause vomiting as soon as they become warm in the stomach.

Burning pains may occur anywhere in the body, but particularly in the head, stomach, abdomen, and chest and along the spine. There is a tendency to bleed easily, and small wounds may bleed bright red blood freely. Nosebleeds are common and often accompany a cold or cough.

What Makes *Phosphorus* Symptoms

Worse: cold or heat (either or both), lying on left or painful side, thunderstorms

Better: massaging or rubbing, cold food and drinks

*Pulsatilla**
Windflower

Pulsatilla is one of the most commonly used medicines for people with acute illnesses of all kinds. Often it is selected primarily because of the patient's emotional nature: those who need *Pulsatilla* tend to have gentle, mild, yielding dispositions along with a desire for attention. Characteristic physical symptoms include lack of thirst, pains that wander from one part of the body to another, and constantly changing symptoms in general. The symptoms are aggravated by heat and improved with slow movement. *Pulsatilla* is commonly indicated for people with colds, coughs, digestive troubles, eye and ear infections, as well as many other conditions.

Vulnerability, weepy sensitivity, and a desire for affection and consolation characterize the *Pulsatilla* personality. The *Pulsatilla* child, for example, becomes clingy, whiny, teary, and fussy. Though she may be fussy and irritable, she is almost never given to full-blown temper tantrums (as inconsolable *Chamomilla* or *Hepar* children are). The *Pulsatilla* patient wants people around her and craves comforting and soothing attention. She seeks sympathy and feels better when she gets it. She may be fearful of being alone or in the dark.

Changeable emotions are typical of people who need *Pulsatilla.* They tend to be moody—happy and laughing one moment, sad and crying the next. They cry easily, even at the thought of pain, and when sick they may break into tears for no apparent reason. They are easily hurt emotionally; receiving slight criticism, being ignored, or hearing loved ones argue may deeply affect them.

**See also* chapters 3 on fever and influenzas, 4 on colds and coughs, 5 on childhood illnesses, 6 on earaches, 8 on digestive problems, 9 on women's health, 10 on men's health, 11 on headaches, and 12 on allergies.

In general, *Pulsatilla* patients are sweet and likable, and they like people to like them. They are sensitive to what others think about them, and they do what they can to please others. They tend to be generous, and they may tell you what you want to hear to get your approval.

The sweet and loving disposition of the *Pulsatilla* patient makes it easy for people to offer comfort and support. In turn, the *Pulsatilla* patient thrives on the attention. There is a tendency to be self-pitying, and the person who is sick may whine, "Why does this always have to happen to me?" or, "Why don't people understand me more?" Offer a little sympathy, however, and she quickly forgets these worries.

These people are often indecisive. They may ask for something but once they get it, they want something else. They are easily led and easily swayed and don't tend to be stubborn.

The physical symptoms of *Pulsatilla* patients are as changeable as the psychological ones. Symptoms shift from one part of the body to another or change character frequently. The pains may appear suddenly and disappear gradually. Sometimes the stools have a different consistency or color with every bowel movement.

Physically, *Pulsatilla* patients are "warm-blooded"; they don't need much clothing and even prefer cold weather. They are sensitive to heat and to warm rooms, and they become less energetic and develop physical symptoms when exposed to heat. They have difficulty sleeping if the room is warm. They thrive in cool, open air, as it relieves many of their symptoms. However, they may get sick from being chilled during warm weather, and they sometimes develop symptoms after eating ice cream.

Slow, gentle motion, especially in the open air, is beneficial to the *Pulsatilla* patient. Walking about slowly often relieves the headache, digestive symptoms, or aches and pains, and it makes the person feel better in general.

Even if they are feverish, *Pulsatilla* patients are rarely thirsty. In fact, during acute illnesses they are usually less thirsty than normal and must be reminded to drink enough liquids.

Pulsatilla is known for body discharges that are thick in character and yellow to green in color. Mucus from a runny nose, phlegm brought up with a cough, and discharges from the eyes, ears, or vagina all have these characteristics. These secretions are produced in large quantity but do not irritate the skin.

The *Pulsatilla* patient often has digestive problems. Her abdomen becomes bloated and sensitive to touch, especially after she's eaten. Digestive symptoms may start shortly after her eating rich or fatty foods, pork, ice cream, fruit, or cold things. She wants something to eat but can't decide what she wants. She may crave foods she can't digest or that make her feel bad. The patient usually is averse to fat, pork, meat, milk, or bread.

What Makes Pulsatilla Symptoms

Worse: warm or closed rooms, foods rich in fat, hot food or drinks, eating, evening, lying on painless side

Better: cool and open air, cold applications, cold food or drinks (though the patient is not thirsty), lying on painful side

*Rhus Toxicodendron**
Poison Ivy

Relief of symptoms by motion is the fundamental characteristic of *Rhus tox.* This applies as much to the various individual symptoms as to those of the person as a whole. In particular, painful joints and muscles hurt when at rest and when first moved, and they get much better as they grow limber during continued motion. In general, the *Rhus tox.* patient is restless and anxious and cannot be comfortable unless she is moving about. She restlessly tosses and turns in bed, and she feels mentally restless and anxious as well.

The restlessness and anxiety make sleep difficult for the *Rhus tox.* patient. Symptoms are generally worse in the evening, as well as during the night, when the patient may also feel more irritable and fearful. In addition, she may be very depressed and may tend to weep easily.

**See also* chapters 3 on fever and influenza, 4 on colds and coughs, 5 on childhood illnesses, 7 on sore throats, 12 on allergies, 13 on skin problems, and 14 on accidents and injuries.

Rhus tox. patients are generally chilly and are aggravated by cold and damp weather. Symptoms worsen if even a single part of the body is uncovered or otherwise becomes cold.

Rhus tox. markedly affects fibrous tissues: joints, tendons, ligaments, and connective tissues. The characteristic pains, worse on first motion and better by continued motion, may be felt during acute illnesses, like the flu, or may be caused by an injury. In fact, even though the pains are better during motion, sustained or vigorous exertion can be difficult for the *Rhus tox.* patients. Symptoms often begin after overexertion—for example, after lifting heavy boxes or working out too strenuously.

The pains in the muscles and joints are achy, sore, or needlelike in character. The joints are stiff and perhaps swollen as well as painful. The pain is usually made worse by cold of any form (cold air, cold baths, or cold applications) and by damp, cold weather. Warmth relieves the symptoms. Firm pressure can also make the painful parts feel better, and *Rhus tox.* backaches feel better when the person is lying on something hard.

As anyone who has had poison ivy knows, *Rhus tox.* strongly affects the skin. Eruptions are red and inflamed and itch terribly, especially after scratching, at night, and from the warmth of the bed. There are usually inflamed blisters with a *Rhus tox.* eruption, ranging in size from tiny pinpoint vesicles on up. The blisters may be filled with clear fluid or with pus, and the eruptions usually ooze. These *Rhus tox.* symptoms are often experienced when people have chicken pox, herpes, and, of course, poison ivy or poison oak.

The *Rhus tox.* patient is usually thirsty, often for cold drinks or milk. Cold drinks, however, may aggravate the symptoms. A peculiar *Rhus tox.* symptom is the presence of a triangular red area at the tip of the tongue.

What Makes *Rhus tox.* Symptoms

Worse: initial motion, prolonged rest, overexertion, cold, cold and damp weather, uncovering, getting wet, night

Better: continued motion, change of position, perspiring, warm applications, warm covering, pressure, rubbing

Sepia*
The Cuttlefish

A lack of vitality, even a sense of lifelessness, is characteristic of *Sepia.* The person feels sluggish and lacks energy. Yet, when she does muster her strength to exercise, she feels much better. Dancing, walking rapidly, or other vigorous exercise improves the person's general condition and many of her specific physical symptoms. The lack of vitality of the *Sepia* person is also evident in her intolerance of cold temperature.

The lifelessness typical of the *Sepia* physical condition may also be apparent in the psychological state. The person becomes withdrawn, emotionally cold, easily angered, and depressed. She may feel an emptiness inside, a sense of indifference or apathy. This may become so strong that she feels indifference or even aversion to her own spouse, children, or siblings. She becomes uninterested in affection and sex, and she may actively dislike lovemaking.

Sepia patients can be moody, feeling sad, gentle, and yielding at one moment, disagreeable, excitable, and stubborn at the next. They are easily offended and can be mean to those around them. They are often averse to company yet may dread being alone. Their defenses are brittle and they weep easily. They are aggravated by efforts to comfort them.

Sepia patients may be so averse to food they cannot stand its smell, and the smell of food may cause intense nausea. They may have a gnawing hunger or a sensation of emptiness in the stomach or abdomen that food does not satisfy. On the other hand, sometimes nausea improves after they've eaten, and they may feel generally better after a meal. *Sepia* patients are often constipated. They tend to crave sour, bitter, pungent, and spicy foods; they may strongly dislike bread, fats, milk, meat, or salt. Eating bread, fats, fruit, milk, pork, or sour foods may make them feel worse.

Sepia patients sometimes experience a sensation of a ball inside

---

See also chapters 5 on childhood illnesses, 9 on women's health, and 13 on skin problems.

the body. They may have this feeling in the throat, abdomen, rectum, or uterus. *Sepia* women may experience a feeling of pressure and bearing down, as if things were protruding from the vagina. When this happens, they feel a strong need to keep the legs crossed to relieve the feeling of pressure and protrusion.

What Makes *Sepia* Symptoms

Worse: cold, 4–6 P.M., morning, menstruation, smelling food, beginning to move, milk, pork, fats, bread, fruit, sour foods, thunderstorms.

Better: dancing, walking rapidly, vigorous exercise, hard pressure, eating

*Silica**
The Chemical Element Flint

"Weakly" might be the best one-word description of people who need *Silica.* During an acute illness a lack of mental and physical stamina prevails, whether the person is normally vigorous or feeble. When he is ill, the *Silica* patient's physiological defenses lack vigor. His symptoms develop slowly and without violence, though he may eventually become very sick.

Often *Silica* patients are basically intelligent and perceptive, but their minds tire easily and become dull, sluggish, and confused. Though they may have trouble thinking and concentrating, they have a tendency to become preoccupied with insignificant details. They doubt their abilities though, if they push themselves, they usually successfully meet a challenge. The *Silica* patient is timid, faint hearted, and yielding. He is not likely to assert his own opinions and generally won't push himself on others. He is happy to be seen and not heard.

---

*See also chapters 4 on colds and coughs, 6 on earaches, 13 on skin problems, and 14 on accidents and injuries.

Despite this passivity, however, he can be stubborn and irritable. He resents interference and withdraws into himself if asked to do something he doesn't want to. He is irritated by attempts to console him. Although nervous and perhaps fidgety, the person who needs *Silica* is not really anxious and is rarely troubled by intense fears.

Silica patients lack physical stamina. They are easily tired and easily chilled. Their hands and feet get cold and can't be warmed. Open air and drafts aggravate this, and like *Hepar* and *Rhus* patients, they may develop symptoms if a single part of the body is uncovered or gets cold. Inflamed parts, however, are not so sensitive to cold as those of *Hepar* patients.

This lack of vitality is also evident in other symptoms. Little wounds tend to become infected, and skin infections are slow to heal, leaving reddened cysts rather than clearing completely. Constipation is common. The body lacks the strength to completely expel the stool, and the stool recedes into the rectum.

Here are some specific symptoms: Swollen lymph nodes occur frequently. Profuse, offensive perspiration, especially on the feet, hands, head, and lower back is distinctive. *Silica* children typically perspire on the back of the head and the neck; the sweat smells sour. These children may also vomit after drinking milk, even breast milk. There may be a sensation as though a splinter or stick were caught in the throat or other inflamed areas. Again, the similarity to *Hepar* is evident, but *Silica* infections, though painful, are not as tender to touch as are those of *Hepar.*

Silica patients may dislike meat and milk. Children may refuse even mother's milk. Though cold food or drinks may make symptoms worse, the patient may have an aversion to warm foods. Thirst may be increased, especially at night.

What Makes *Silica* Symptoms

Worse: cold, open air, winter, damp weather, uncovering, coldness or uncovering of a single part of the body, getting the feet wet, cold food or drinks, lying on the painful side, suppressed perspiration, eating

Better: warmth

Sulphur*
The Chemical Element†

Sulphur is one of the most commonly prescribed homeopathic medicines for chronically ill people. It is only occasionally prescribed for acute illness, but it should be considered during fevers, skin conditions, and a variety of other conditions whenever the overall *Sulphur* picture is present.

Sulphur patients are usually invigorated by cold weather and by being in the open air. They feel worse when it is warm, in warm rooms, and in warm beds. Along with this internal heat, burning pains and discharges that cause burning discomfort are often experienced. The eyes, ears, nose, throat, stomach, anus, or the top of the head may burn. Most characteristically, the soles of the feet burn. The *Sulphur* patient may need to stick the feet or hands out of the covers. The lips and other mucous membranes are red and dry. Their skin in general, and particularly the face, is reddened.

Discharges, whether from the nose, skin, eyes, ears or elsewhere, are likely to have an offensive odor. The breath, stool, and sweat also smell bad. Yet the patient is often unaware of his odor, though at the same time he may be overly sensitive to other odors around him. Some *Sulphur* patients find their own odor extremely offensive, even after they bathe. Often the patient doesn't like to wash, and bathing may aggravate some of his symptoms, especially those on the skin.

Suphur patients are often robust and emotionally thick-skinned; they are less emotionally sensitive than patients who need medicines such as *Pulsatilla* or *Nux vomica*. When they are acutely ill, they may be impatient, hurried, and quick tempered. Yet they tend to be lazy and averse to business or any systematic work. They become sloppy and disorganized and allow home and work environments to become messy. The disorder doesn't bother them, however, since they claim to know where everything is when they

---

See also chapters 7 on sure throats, 10 on men's health, 12 on allergies, and 13 on skin problems.

†*Sulphur* should not be given immediately after *Calcarea*.

need it. People who need *Sulphur* are "pack rats," keeping old possessions because of the special meaning each has. The *Sulphur* patient's appearance is also messy. His clothes are disheveled and dirty and his hair is unkempt.

While he ignores his external environment, the *Sulphur* patient may become obsessed with abstract concepts, religious or philosophical issues, or other subjects that do not have definitive answers. He may become preoccupied with obscure facts and details or with grand pipe-dreams, though he is often unproductive.

Sulphur children are self-centered and demanding. They may hoard toys they aren't using, or concern themselves only with how things affect them, while ignoring the needs of others. They are inquisitive, especially asking questions that cannot be answered.

Sulphur is known for a number of digestive symptoms. One distinctive symptom is an empty sensation in the stomach that may or may not be associated with hunger. Often around 11 A.M. the patient has a ravenous appetite that comes on suddenly and cannot be satisfied. He often suffers indigestion after eating. Early in the morning he may be driven out of bed by a powerful, sudden urge to have a bowel movement. He tends to like strong-tasting foods and may crave spicy foods, sweets, fatty foods, and alcohol. He may also be averse to milk, meat, sweets, and fats; bread, cold food or drinks, fats, sweets, milk, or even the sight of food may aggravate symptoms.

The *Sulphur* patient is usually quite thirsty. He may prefer warm drinks, which may indeed make his symptoms better.

The *Sulphur* patient may be unable to get to sleep before midnight, or he may be troubled by waking up too early (3 A.M. or somewhat later is common). He is likely to feel unusually lethargic after he has overslept.

Sulphur is commonly prescribed for a wide variety of skin conditions, and rashes or other skin eruptions may accompany any condition for which the medicine is indicated. Itching is usually intense and is worse at night in warmth, and in warm beds. Scratching may relieve this temporarily but often results in increased itching and burning.

Typically, people who need *Sulphur* experience more complaints on the left than right side of the body.

What Makes *Sulphur* Symptoms

Worse: warmth, warm rooms, warmth of the bed, cold air, left side, 11 A.M., standing, washing, scratching, long sleep, changeable weather.

Better: open air, warm drinks

PART
4

Homeopathic
Resources

Homeopathic Organizations

National Center for Homoeopathy
1500 Massachusetts Avenue, NW
Washington, DC 20005

American Institute of Homoeopathy
1500 Massachusetts Avenue, NW
Washington, DC 20005

United States Homeopathic Association
6560 Backlick Road
Springfield, VA 22150

International Foundation for Homeopathy
1141 NW Market Street
Seattle, WA 98107

Liga Medicorm Homoeopathica Internationalis
(The International League for Homoeopathic Medicine)
P.O. Box 66
A. B. Bloemendaal, The Netherlands

Pan-American Homeopathic Medical Congress
Francisco del Paso y Troncoso Edificio 166
Entrada D. Unidad Kennedy
Mexico 9, D.F.

British Homoeopathic Association
27A Devonshire Street
London, W1N 1RJ, England

Sources of Homeopathic Medicines

The following are some of the major sources of homeopathic medicines. There are many other pharmacies and health food stores that sell homeopathic medicines. If you do not know of one nearby, all of the following pharmacies and homeopathic businesses offer active and reliable mail-order services. They also sell homeopathic home medicine kits. We highly recommend obtaining such a kit since it is problematic to have to send away for medicines when you or someone close to you needs homeopathic care now. It is also considerably cheaper to purchase a kit than to buy medicines individually.

Boericke and Tafel, Inc.
1011 Arch Street
Philadelphia, PA 19107

John A. Bornemann and Sons
1208 Amosland Road
Norwood, PA 19074

Ehrhart and Karl, Inc.
17 N Wabash Avenue
Chicago, IL 60602

HRI-Dolisos
6125 Tropicana Avenue
Las Vegas, NV 89103

Homeopathic Educational Services
2124 Kittredge Street
Berkeley, CA 94704

Humphreys Pharmacal Company*
63 Meadow Road
Rutherford, NJ 07070

Luyties Pharmacal Company
4200 Laclede Avenue
St. Louis, MO 63108

Standard Homeopathic Pharmacy
204-210 W 131st Street
Los Angeles, CA 90061

Washington Homeopathic Pharmacy
4914 Delray Avenue
Bethesda, MD 20814

---

*These pharmacies primarily sell combination medicines.

Homeopathic Books and Tapes

Homeopathic Educational Services
2124 Kittredge Street
Berkeley, CA 94704
(This center also sells cassette tapes on homeopathic subjects and homeopathic medicine kits, and general information on homeopathy is also available)

Yes! Inc. Bookshop
1035 Thirty-first Street, NW
Washington, DC 20007

Glossary

Allopathy: The homeopathic term for conventional medicine. "Allos" in Greek means "other than" or "different from" and "pathy" means "disease" or "suffering." Allopathic medicine refers to the practice of prescribing pharmaceuticals that are chosen simply because they diminish symptoms, often because they are antagonistic to the disease process.

Antidote: A substance or experience that slows, stops or reverses the curative action of a homeopathic medicine.

Casetaking: The interview process used in homeopathy to determine the correct homeopathic medicine.

Common symptoms: Those symptoms that people typically experience with a specific disease (e.g., jaundice and lack of appetite during hepetitis). These symptoms are the least important in determining the correct homeopathic medicine for the individual.

Constitution: The overall health of the person as determined by his/her heredity, life history, lifestyle, environment, and past treatments.

Constitutional treatment: Treatment that is determined by a careful assessment of a person's constitution and present total symptomatology in an effort to stimulate the person's inner healing most deeply.

Cure: A profound overall improvement in health in which the individual achieves a sense of physical, emotional and mental freedom.

Drug picture: The essential characteristics of a homeopathic medicine's action compiled from collected provings, accounts of poisonings, and clinical experience. Also referred to as "essence of a medicine" or a "medicine's essence."

General symptoms: Those symptoms which pertain to the person as a whole, including all psychological symptoms and those physical symptoms in which the whole body is affected (e.g. energy level, restlessness, sensitivity to cold, tiredness in the morning). Because these symptoms are representations of the body's overall response, they are considered deeper symptoms and thus are particularly important in choosing the correct homeopathic medicine.

Globules: Pellet-sized sugar pills on which the potentized solution is dropped (larger than granules).

Granules: Small grain of sand-sized sugar pills on which the potentized solution is dropped (smaller than globules).

Healing crisis: A common experience of those who use homeopathic medicines to treat chronic conditions and some acute illnesses in which some more external symptoms initially get worse in the process of cure. (Sometimes referred to by Homeopaths as "aggravation" of symptoms.)

Hering's Laws of Cure: First described by Constantine Hering (1800– 1880), these principles define the changes in symptoms that should be observed during a genuine curative response to treatment. The three components are 1) healing proceeds from the deepest parts within the organism necessary for survival and growth extending outward to the most superficial parts; 2) healing proceeds from the top of the person to the bottom; and 3) healing proceeds in reverse order of the symptoms' appearance in the person.

Law of similars: The fundamental tenet of homeopathy that states that a substance which causes a set of symptoms in a healthy person acts as a curative medicine when given to sick people who have its similar symptoms.

Materia medica: Taken from Latin, meaning "materials of medicines." Homeopathic *materia medicas* are books that list the medicines used and the detailed indications for their application.

Modality: A circumstance that makes a person's overall health or a specific symptom better or worse (e.g. in weakness worse in the morning or headache better by cold applications, "worse in the morning" and "better by cold applications" are the modalities).

Nosode: A homeopathic medicine made of material taken from diseased material, such as bacteria, viruses, and pus.

Palliation of symptoms: The temporary relief of symptoms without actually curing the disease from which they originated.

Particular symptoms: Those symptoms which are local to a specific area of the body (e.g. a throbbing pain in the head, a burning pain in the stomach, an itching on the scalp).

Polychrest: A homeopathic medicine that has many uses.

Potency: The term used in homeopathy to describe the number of times a substance has been diluted and succussed (shaken) according to the strict rules of the *Homoeopathic Pharmacopeia*. When an "x" is written after a number (as in 6x, 30x), it refers to the number of times one part of a medicine was diluted with nine parts of the dilutant (usually distilled water). When a "c" is written after a number (as in 6c, 30c), this refers to the number of times one part of a medicine was diluted with 99 parts of dilutant. When "lm" is written after a number (as in 6lm, 30lm), this refers to the number of times one part of a medicine was diluted with 50,000 parts of dilutant.

Potentization: The pharmaceutical process of repeated dilution with succussion (vigorous shaking) by which the homeopathic medicines are prepared.

Proving: The procedure for giving doses of a substance to healthy subjects in order to find what it causes in overdose and thus what it has the capacity to cure when given to ill people in potentized dose.

Repertory: A valuable homeopathic text that is an index of symptoms and a listing of those medicines which have been found to cause and/or cure specific symptoms.

Repertorization: The process of determining the correct medicine for the person by noting their characteristic symptoms, by finding in a repertory what substances cause these symptoms, by determining what substances cause the greatest number of symptoms, and then by selecting the one substance that most accurately fits the whole person.

Rubric: A symptom that is listed in a repertory.

Similia: A Greek word meaning "similar;" used in reference to the law of similars.

Simillimum: The medicine most similar to the person's totality of symptoms.

Strange, rare and peculiar symptoms: These are symptoms that are unusual in people or are contradictory to what most people experience with a similar illness.

Succussion: An integral part of the homeopathic pharmaceutical process in which a medicinal substance is diluted in distilled water and is vigorously shaken by striking it against a firm surface.

Suppression of symptoms: To treat symptoms in such a way that they disappear but other more serious symptoms manifest.

Symptoms: Observable or felt changes in the physical, emotional or mental condition of a person that limit optimal health. Homeopaths believe that symptoms represent efforts of the organism to deal with an internal or external stress.

Vis medicatrix naturae: The inherent healing power of the organism which automatically works in a self-regulating, self-organizing capacity to re-establish health, often creating various symptoms as its way to externalizing the stress to inner processes.

Suggested Homeopathic Readings

The following are some of the most important books in homeopathic medicine. There are many other good and helpful books in the field not listed here. Contact the sources of homeopathic books mentioned for more information on them.

Introductory and Self-Care Books

Coulter, Harris L., Ph.D. *Homoeopathic Medicine.* St. Louis: Formur, 1972.

Gibson, D. M., M.D. *First Aid Homoeopathy in Accidents and Injuries.* London: British Homoeopathic Association.

Panos, Maesimund, M.D., and Jane Heimlich. *Homeopathic Medicine at Home.* Los Angeles: J. P. Tarcher, 1980.

Santwani, M. T., M.D. *Common Ailments of Children and their Homoeopathic Treatment.* New Delhi: Jain, 1979.

Shadman, Alonzo, M.D. *Who is Your Doctor and Why.* 1958. Reprint. New Canaan, CT: Keats, 1980.

Shepherd, Dorothy, M.D. *Homoeopathy for the First Aider.* Essex, England: Health Sciences, 1945.

Smith, Trevor, M.D. *Homoeopathic Medicine: A Doctor's Guide to Remedies for Common Ailments.* New York: Thorsons, 1983.

_____ . *A Woman's Guide to Homoeopathic Medicine.* New York: Thorsons, 1984.

Vithoulkas, George. *Homeopathy: Medicine of the New Man.* New York: Arco, 1979.

Weiner, Michael, Ph.D., and Kathleen Goss. *The Complete Book of Homeopathy.* New York: Bantam, 1981.

Philosophy, Methodology and Research

Coulter, Harris, Ph.D. *Homoeopathic Science and Modern Medicine: The Physics of Healing with Microdoses.* Berkeley: North Atlantic, 1981.

Crews, Richard, M.D. *Introductory Workbook in Homeopathy.* Berkeley: Homeopathic Educational Services, 1980.

Dhawale, M. L., M.D. *Principles and Practice of Homoeopathy.* Bombay: D. K. Homoeopathic Corporation, 1967.

Hahnemann, Samuel, M.D. *Organon of Medicine.* 1842. Reprint. Los Angeles: J. P. Tarcher, 1982.

Kent, James T., M.D. *Lectures on Homoeopathic Philosophy.* 1900. Reprint. Berkeley: North Atlantic, 1979.

Roberts, H. A., M.D. *The Principles and Art of Cure by Homoeopathy.* Essex, England: Health Sciences, 1942.

Ullman, Dana, M.P.H. *Monograph on Homeopathic Research.* Berkeley: Homeopathic Educational Services, 1981.

Vithoulkas, George. *The Science of Homeopathy.* New York: Grove, 1979.

Wright, Elizabeth, M.D. (Elizabeth Wright Hubbard). *A Brief Study Course in Homoeopathy.* St. Louis: Formur, 1977.

Whitmont, Edward C., M.D. *Psyche and Substance: Essays on Homeopathy in the Light of Jungian Psychology.* Berkeley: North Atlantic, 1980.

History of Homeopathy

Coulter, Harris L., Ph.D. *Divided Legacy: A History of the Schism in Medical Thought.* Vol. 1, *The Patterns Emerge: Hippocrates to Paracelsus.* (350 B.C.–1600 A.D.). Vol. 2, *Progress and Regress: J. B. Helmont to Claude Bernard* (1600–1850). Washington, DC: Wehawken Books, 1977 and 1975. Volume III: *The Conflict Between Homoeopathy and the American Medical Association: Science and Ethics in American Medicine* (1800–1914). Berkeley: North Atlantic Books, 1981.

————. *Homoeopathic Influences in 19th Century Allopathic Therapeutics.* St. Louis: Formur, 1977.

Grossinger, Richard, Ph.D. *Planet Medicine: From Stone Age Shaminism to Post-Industrial Healing.* Boulder: Shambhala, 1982.

Veterinary Homeopathy

MacLeod, George, M.R.C.V.S., D.V.S.M., *The Homoeopathic Treatment of Dogs.* London: Homoeopathic Development Foundation, 1983.

_____ . *Veterinary Materia Medica with Repertory.* Essex, England: Health Sciences, 1983.

_____ . *Treatment of Horses by Homoeopathy.* Essex, England: Health Sciences, 1981.

Pitcairn, Richard H., D.V.M., Ph.D. and Susan Pitcairn, M.A., *Natural Health for Dogs and Cats.* Emmaus, PA: Rodale, 1982.

Materia Medicas and Repertories

Allen, H. C., M.D. *Keynotes and Characteristics of the Materia Medica with Nosodes.* New Delhi: Jain.

Baker, Wyrth Post, M.D. (Wyrth Post Baker), Allen Neiswander, M.D., and W. W. Young, M.D. *Introduction to Homeotherapeutics.* Washington, DC: American Institute of Homoeopathy, 1974.

Boericke, William, M.D. *Pocket Manual of Materia Medica with Repertory.* 1936. Reprint. New Delhi: Jain, 1982.

Clarke, John, M.D. *Dictionary of Practical Materia Medica.* 3 vols. 1900. Reprint. Essex, England: Health Sciences, 1962.

Farrington, E. A., M.D. *Clinical Materia Medica.* 1887. Reprint. Calcutta: Ringer, 1982.

Hering, Constantine, M.D. *Guiding Symptoms of Our Materia Medica.* 1879. Reprint. New Delhi: Jain, 1977.

Kent, James, M.D. *Lectures on Homoeopathic Materia Medica.* 1904. Reprint. New Delhi: Jain, 1974.

_____ . *Repertory of Homoeopathic Materia Medica.* 1877. Reprint. New Delhi: Jain, 1982.

Nash, E. B., M.D. *Leaders in Homoeopathic Therapeutics.* 1898. Reprint. New Delhi: Jain, 1983.

Tyler, Margaret, M.D. *Drug Pictures.* Essex, England: Health Sciences, 1952.

Wheeler, Charles, M.D. *An Introduction to the Principles and Practice of Homoepoathy.* Essex, England: Health Sciences, 1948.

References

Abramowicz, Mark (ed.). *The Medical Letter,* 56 Harrison, New Rochelle, New York 10801.

Bach, Edward, and F. J. Wheeler. *The Bach Flower Remedies.* New Canaan, CT: Keats, 1977.

Barnard, G. P., and James Stephenson. "Microdose Paradox: A New Biophysical Concept," *Journal of the American Institute of Homoeopathy* 60 (September, 1967). In *Monograph. See* Ullman, 1980.

_____ . "Fresh Evidence for a Biophysical Field," *Journal of the American Institute of Homoeopathy* 62 (April, 1969) 73–85. In *Monograph. See* Ullman, 1980.

Barness, Lewis A. *Manual of Pediatric Physical Diagnosis.* Chicago: Year Book Medical Publishers, 1981.

Bierman, June, and Barbara Toohey. *The Woman's Holistic Headache Relief Book.* Los Angeles: J. P. Tarcher, 1979.

Boericke, William, and W. A. Dewey. *Twelve Tissue Salts.* New Delhi: Indian Books and Periodicals. 1914. Reprint.

Boiron, Jean, Jacky Abecassis, and Philippe Belon. *Aspects of Research in Homeopathy.* Lyon, France: Boiron, 1983.

Boyd, Linn. *The Simile in Medicine.* Philadelphia: Boericke and Tafel, 1936.

Bradford, Thomas Lindsay. *The Logic of Figures or Comparative Results of Homoeopathic and Other Treatments.* Philadelphia: Boericke and Tafel, 1900.

Carroll, David. *The Complete Book of Natural Medicines.* New York: Summitt, 1980.

Cattell, J. McKean (ed.). *Science* 72 (1930): 526.

Cave, Ray (ed.). "Those Overworked Medical Drugs," *Time* (August 17, 1981).

Coulter, Harris L. *Divided Legacy: A History of the Schism in Medical Thought.* Vol. 1, *The Patterns Emerge: Hippocrates to Paracelsus (350 B.C.–1600 A.D.).* Vol. 2, *Progress and Regress: J. B. Helmont to Claude Bernard (1600–1850).* Washington, DC: Wehawken, 1975, 1977. Vol. 3, *The Conflict Between Homoeopathy and the American Medical Association: Science and Ethics in American Medicine (1800–1914).* Berkeley: North Atlantic, 1981.

―――― . *Homoeopathic Science and Modern Medicine: The Physics of Healing with Microdoses.* Berkeley: North Atlantic, 1981.

Diamont, M., et. al. "Abuse and Time of Use of Antibiotics in Acute Otitis Media." *Archives in Otolaryngology* 100 (1974): 226–32.

Dubos, Rene. Introduction in *Anatomy of an Illness* by Norman Cousins, 23, New York: W. W. Norton, 1979.

Evans, Starling, and Lovatt Evans. *Principles of Human Physiology* 14th edition. London: J & A Churchill, 1968.

Feinbloom, Richard L. and Boston Children's Medical Center. *Child Health Encyclopedia,* New York: Dell, 1975.

Ferguson, Tom (ed.). *Medical Self-Care: Access to Health Tools.* New York: Summitt, 1980.

―――― . *Medical Self-Care,.* P. O. Box 717, Inverness, CA. 94937.

Fishman, Mark C., Andrew R. Hoffman, Richard D. Klausner, Stanley G. Rockson, and Malcolm S. Thaler. *Medicine.* Philadelphia, J. B. Lippincott, 1981.

Fisher, Peter and Ifor Capel. "The Treatment of Experimental Lead Intoxication in Rats by Penicillamine and Plumbum (200c)—A Controlled Trial." *Journal of Ultramolecular Medicine* 1 (1983): 30–31. In *Monograph. See* Ullman, 1980.

Florey, Sir Howard W. *British Medical Journal,* (1943):654.

Galpin, Jeffrey E. (ed.). "Does Zinc Have an Effect on the Common Cold?" *Infectious Disease Alert,* 3, no. 12 (1984).

Gibson, R. G., Shiela L. M. Gibson, A. D. MacNeill, and W. Watson. "Homoeopathic Therapy in Rheumatoid Arthritis: Evaluation by Double-Blind Clinical Therapeutic Trial." *British Journal of Clinical Pharmacology,* (May, 1980): 453–459.

Graedon, Joe. *The People's Pharmacy-2.* New York: Avon, 1980.

Hahnemann, Samuel. *Lesser Writings.* New York: Radde, 1852.

Hastings, Arthur, James Fadiman, and James Gordon. *Health for the Whole Person.* New York: Bantam, 1980.

Hockelman, R. A., et. al. *Principles of Pediatrics,* New York: McGraw-Hill, 1978.

Hudak, Carolyn M., Paul M. Redstone, Nancy L. Hokanson, and Irene E. Suzuki. *Clinical Protocols.* Philadelphia: J. B. Lippincott, 1976.

Jaffe, Dennis. *Healing From Within.* New York: Bantam, 1982.

Kluger, Matthew J. "Fever and Survival," *Science,* 188 (April, 1975):166–168.

———. "Fever," *Pediatrics* 66 (November, 1980): 720–724.

Kluger, Matthew J., and Barbara A. Rothenburg. "Fever and Reduced Iron: Their Interaction as a Host Defense Response to Bacterial Infection." *Science* 203 (January 26, 1979): 374–376.

———. "Fever, Trace Metals, and Disease." In *Fever,* edited by J. M. Lipton, New York: Raven, 1980.

Krupp, Marcus A., and Milton J. Chatton. *Current Medical Diagnosis and Treatment.* Los Altos, CA: Lange, 1982.

Lappe, Marc. *Germs That Won't Die.* New York: Anchor, 1982.

Levin, Alan Scott, and Merla Zellerbach. *The Type 1/Type 2 Allergy Relief Program.* Los Angeles: J. P. Tarcher, 1983.

McHugh, Paul. "Rattler!" *San Francisco Magazine* (May, 1982): 58–63.

Norton, Ruth (ed.). "Challenge of a Painful Pox." *Acute Care Medicine* 1, 3 (1984): 12–28.

Office of Technology Assessment. *Assessing the Efficacy and Safety of Medical Technologies.* Washington, DC: Government Printing Office, 1978.

Pantell, Robert H., James F. Fries, and Donald M. Vickery. *Taking Care of Your Child.* Reading, MA: Addison-Wesley, 1982.

Paradise, J. L. "Otitis Media in Infants and Children." *Pediatrics* 65, no. 5 (1980): 917.

Paterson, John. "Report on Mustard Gas Experiments." *British Homoeopathic Journal.* 33, no. 1, (1943).

Pelletier, Kenneth R. *Holistic Medicine: From Stress to Optimum Health.* New York: Delacorte/Lawrence, 1979.

———. *Mind as Healer, Mind as Slayer* New York: Delacorte/Lawrence, 1977.

Ritz, Sandra. "Bladder Infections." *Medical Self-Care* (Spring, 1981): 9–14.

Sehnert, Keith. *How to Be Your Own Doctor (Sometimes).* New York: Grosset & Dunlap, 1975.

Selye, Hans. *The Stress of Life.* New York: McGraw-Hill, 1978, 12–13.

Smith, Lendon. *The Encyclopedia of Baby & Child Care.* New York: Warner, 1980.

Stephenson, James. "A Review of Investigations into the Action of Substances in Dilutions Greater than 1 Times 10 (micro-dilutions)." *Journal of the American Institute of Homoeopathy* (November, 1955): 327–335. In *Monograph. See* Ullman, 1980.

———. "A Literature Survey of the Properties of High Dilutions." *Journal of the American Institute of Homoeopathy.* (September, 1961): 144–151. In *Monograph. See* Ullman, 1980.

———. "Field Pharmacology: An Historical Review." *Journal of The American Institute of Homoeopathy.* (February, 1964). In *Monograph. See* Ullman, 1980.

Tiller, William. "A Rationale for the Homeopathic Law of Similars." *Journal of Homeopathic Practice* 2, no. 1, (1979): 48–52. In *Monograph. See* Ullman, 1980.

Ullman, Dana (ed.). *Monograph on Homeopathic Research.* Berkeley: Homeopathic Educational Services, 1980.

Van Buchen, F. L., et al. "Therapy of Acute Ototis Media: Myringotomy, Antibiotics, or Neither?" *Lancet,* 2, no. 8252 (1981): 883–887.

Vickery, Donald M., and James F. Fries. *Take Care of Yourself: A Consumer's Guide to Medical Care.* Reading, MA: Addison-Wesley, 1978.

Vithoulkas, George. *The Science of Homeopathy.* New York: Grove, 1979.

Whitmont, Edward C. *Psyche and Substance: Essays on Homeopathy in the Light of Jungian Psychology.* Berkeley: North Atlantic, 1980.

Index